Dedicated to TAL, AUGIE AND GEORGE:

the shape of my heart.

You are amazing grace. You are a precious jewel.
You—special miraculous, unrepeatable,
fragile, fearful, tender, lost,
sparkling ruby emerald
jewel rainbow splendor
person.
~Joan Baez

Shine on!
2017

He's got to make his own mistakes
And learn to mend the mess he makes
He's old enough to know what's right
And young enough not to choose it
~Rush, *New World Man*

Special Thanks to these members of MY VILLAGE
who helped bring this book to life:

Christie Lane Thomas, Rita Mailander, Dr. Jeanie Engelbert,
Kim Dreiling, Stephanie Cozart, Gwendolyn Harmsen, Lynda
Schroer, Sara Evert, Jennifer Biltoft, Annette Lane Hartbarger,
Stephen Bridges, Jessica Rettig, Kim Stephan Hightower and all
the teenagers and parents who so generously shared your
stories, struggles and lives with me.

Mike and Marcia Lane, who were saddled with the job of raising a
lunatic like me. Thank you for teaching me girls can do anything.

James Andrew Bridges, my student, teacher, friend and
personal Buddha, who has been there every step of the way.

Table of Contents

IN THE THIRD RING:
THE UNBELIEVABLE TRANSFORMATION OF VIGILANT PARENTS

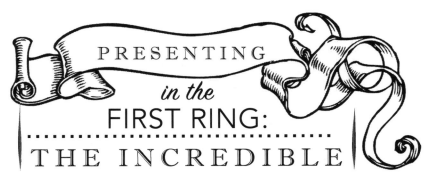

PRESENTING
in the
FIRST RING:
THE INCREDIBLE
BALANCING ACT
of PARENTING
TEENAGERS

Preface

I Love Teenagers:
Catcher in the Rye Parenting

What I have to do, I have to catch everybody if they start to go over the cliff—
I mean if they're running and they don't look where they're going
I have to come out from somewhere and catch them.
That's all I do all day. I'd just be the catcher in the rye and all.
I know it's crazy, but that's the only thing I'd really like to be.
~J.D. Salinger, *The Catcher in the Rye*

I LOVE TEENAGERS. I need to start with this, because I am going to say horrible things about them. Raising teenagers sucks. But this is also true: I love them. I adore teenagers in exactly the same way most people love toddlers. They really are so very much the same (as we'll discuss at greater length in future chapters). Adolescents—like toddlers—are goofy and silly and awkward in their own bodies. They are easily confused and constantly distracted. They fall down a lot. They are prone to temper tantrums. They overreact and over-celebrate and if you catch them in the right mood, they have an overflow of love to share. They say passionate, ridiculous things. I love teenagers and I long to help them when they are in trouble. I want to stand at the edge of Holden Caulfield's crazy cliff and catch them all.

PokeMom poʊˈkeɪ ˈmɑm

An interactive, free to play, location-based reality game in which teenagers roam the lands and a player's (parent's) battle cry is, "Gotta save 'em all!"

This Catcher in the Rye Complex began even before I started teaching high school, before my own children morphed into difficult teenagers, probably somewhere around the time I became a teen in turmoil myself. Young people get lost—go over the cliff, unravel, drift away—in a million ways. If you're a parent, I don't have to tell you; a long list of real predators keeps us all awake at night. Take your pick of worries (or perhaps your progeny will choose for you): everything from good old-fashioned sex, drugs and rock-and-roll to newfangled technology threatens our hormonal offspring. If you are like me, you may be most freaked out by the memories of your own misspent youth. Teenagers are difficult and they are vulnerable, but they are also full of hope.

They are full of hope and they can't help it. It is their lot in life. Teenagers—even when they adopt attitudes of contempt and threaten to grow bitter before their time—believe in the future. Anything is possible as far as they know. Even if it scares them, they look into the next several decades and imagine what might be. They don't see broken dreams or complicated relationships or student loan debt. At 14 and 16 and even 22 they look into the future and see themselves as professional athletes, NASCAR drivers, magicians, fighter pilots, Nobel laureates, artists and activists. They believe—really, really believe, and nothing the cynical adult world does can shake them of the notion—that they can make better happen. That they will change the world. It's nice to spend time with people who have this attitude.

Don't get me wrong; teenagers frustrate me and disappoint me every day. They're so *adolescent* all the time. And—like toddlers—they are so vulnerable! The journey toward adulthood can lead our kids into dangerous territory. Once in a while, despite their youth and natural enthusiasm, one of these adolescents gets lost in the forest of despair. She loses hope. He forgets feelings are temporary. And before we can help them find their way to a clearing (where they can breathe and see and feel okay again) they choose to leave us. Some of the young people I cared about got lost. Some of the teenagers I tried to help didn't make it; some went astray without me even guessing anything was wrong. Some of them have committed suicide or made reckless choices that killed them. Many others have strayed, stood on the edge of that cliff and found their way back. These happy stories we celebrate with a metaphorical fatted calf because those who were lost are found.

Adolescents have a biological imperative to act recklessly. They are quite literally in the midst of identity crisis and it's their job to muck their way through and make the best of it: physically, emotionally and socially. If they don't, their beautiful, authentic identities will never fully mature. A lot of young people simply must run at full speed toward the cliff. I understand this mandate and I want to let them run. But by God, I'd like to catch them before they go over the edge. I know why sprinting toward danger feels so right at their age. When they play with fire, they forge their adult selves. Only when they push limits, test theories, question authority and tilt at windmills can young people become the adults we dream they will be. I also know how wrong things can go, how lost kids can get, and how quickly adolescent angst can send happy families right over the edge.

I care, of course, because it's personal. Like Holden, I've conflated the youngsters with my own lost self. My fantasy really ends with someone swooping in and rewriting history, saving my adolescence from the edge of a terrible cliff. If I shine a light of hope for teenagers or their parents, maybe I'll illuminate my own way out of the darkness. Like most loving parents, my husband and I started our little family with full hearts and the best intentions. Somehow—in spite of our flaws, foibles and wicked ways—we trusted we had the right stuff to raise a couple of human beings. We turned our gaze toward the Divine, read a lot of books, relied on family and friends. We were blessed beyond our wildest dreams with two healthy, beautiful boys. We expected the teenaged years to be rough, but we were confident we would rise to the challenge. For many years, our family ups and downs were bearable and life was pretty sweet. And then almost suddenly (but also gradually, slowly, like the drip of a torturous faucet) we lost our way. Our children turned into emotional, over-sensitive, brooding, irrational, spiteful creatures. It seemed too early to be puberty—so emotional at 11 years old!—and it took us by surprise. Before we knew what was happening (before we could consult the proper parenting manuals), we were in it. Simultaneously, I was spending my days with high school students. I sometimes described my job as, "arguing with teenagers and banging my head against the wall all day long," but I managed to teach them how to read a little better and write decent essays. I also got to know my students pretty well, and because they were a few years ahead of our boys, I started taking notes.

I observed some champion parenting. I saw adults make choices and take actions that saved their children and I saw these children blossom into responsible adulthood. I also observed how adults, including me, let our teenagers down. This job of ours—this parenting of teenagers—is painful, personal and absolutely disorienting. Professionals and experts call adolescence a great "disruption" to the life of a family. No kidding. Even those of us who know better—we with training or education or personal vows to be better than our own parents—fall right through the rabbit hole after our kids. Everything gets topsy-turvy. Logic goes out the window. All bets are off. Pretty soon we find ourselves immersed in power struggles and all the eye-rolling sends us right over the edge into some awfully bad parenting decisions. Although I certainly do not have all the answers, my experience and research have taught me we can change this course. If we meet them with open eyes, strong arms and full hearts, we can help teenagers grow up.

Anyone who has seen me in the full throes of losing my cool will attest I am not a parenting or child development expert. Much of my very own parenting and teaching have been messy and imperfect and marked far more by failure than grace. But I am almost certain what I have to tell you is important. I think you will want to hear it. If you are raising teenagers, I think it may even be vital that you hear it. Like most of us, I am balancing on a high wire strung between good intentions and bad habits, between things I know are true and things that make me doubt everything. Among a smattering of degrees I feel are mostly decorative, however, I earned one I believe applies. Ladies and Gentlemen, allow me to present my PhD in Keepin' it Real. Mine is wisdom learned in the trenches also known as high school English class. These are lessons learned in desperation. Few things are so humbling as realizing your clever lesson on subordinate clauses matters nothing at all to a teenager struggling to find her place in the world, keep her skin clear, or gain the attention of that cute guy back in the corner. High school students stand on the precipice of leaving the nest and starting lives on their own. They are at a unique moment in time when they crave independence and boundaries simultaneously, often in equal measure. They are dizzyingly close to becoming the adults they will soon be and yet they are light years away. They are difficult, rebellious, confused, brilliant, impetuous, impulsive, prone to drama, and really, really stupid.

It is a beautiful mystery how many of my former students are now doing wonderfully well regardless of the parenting they received. The human spirit is invincible; we thrive in rocky soil; we all shine on (like the moon and the stars and the sun). I do believe, however, that parents can make a difference. I believe we have the power to give our children a strong foundation and a view of the world which can help them become the best versions of themselves. Surely we can strive to do no harm to the miracle-people we brought onto the planet.

What I have to tell you is based on years of very real, very raw relationships with teenagers. Here are stories of my own spectacular failures as my children turned into people I did not recognize, who suddenly spit venom at me when I entered a room. Even more importantly, my findings are also based on interviews with parents and teenagers, the latest neuroscience research on adolescence, and tried-and-true theories of family systems. Raising teenagers into responsible adulthood is a hardscrabble, often ugly process. Raising teenagers, I will remind you again and again, is not for the faint of heart. It might threaten to destroy you, your family and everything you hold dear. But raising adolescents to adulthood can also be the richest and most redeeming thing you have ever done. I will share a practical approach to helping our kids (and ourselves!) from getting truly lost. The family journey is by definition imperfect and riddled with failures and mistakes. We do best to admit this messiness and stay committed to our children. We will screw up, because we are flawed people ourselves, but we must not give up. Along the way, let's remember how much we really do love our full-of-hope, vulnerable teenagers.

A Note to Modern Families:

It doesn't matter what your family looks like. Married, single, divorced, "it's complicated:" if you care about a young person on the journey toward adulthood, the tips and tools I have learned from observing champion parents can help. There is no rule book, no silver bullet, no owner's manual for parenting. It's a constant struggle to retain balance on the high wire of raising adolescents. We face all manner of impediments. The ability to detach from the fray, to know, protect and honor our children, to find that precarious balance, can help all of us who care about teenagers, regardless of the shape our family happens to take.

-

Chapter One

Beyond Mama Bear:
Why We Need New Role Models

*Justice does not help those who slumber
but helps only those who are vigilant.*
~Mahatma Gandhi

MAMA BEAR HIBERNATES (AND SO DO WE).

Mama Bear is a great role model for parents of little kids but a dangerous example for parents of teenagers. We're all familiar with the archetype; Mama Bear justifies our slightly crazy parental instincts when our children are small. When we're working to keep innocent cubs safe from harm, Mama Bear makes sense: strong, smart, sassy, sure of herself, guided by pure animal instinct. All of us have "Mama Bear" moments: the dad who leaps to yank a toddler away from speeding cars; the mother who can identify a real cry of trouble three blocks away; the parent who feels an out-of-nowhere urge to yell at menacing big kids on the playground. Yes, we share Mama Bear's instincts to protect our brood. When we pull a toddler away from a hot stove or jolt from our sleep because something feels *not right*, Mama Bear makes sense to us.

Then puberty hits. Our darling children are replaced by strangers with terrible language, weird clothes, bad habits and lousy attitudes. And where is Mama Bear now? Now that her cubs are almost grown, somewhat independent, able to sort of make their way in the world? She's asleep on the job. Hibernating. Checked out. Mama Bear goes to sleep just as her babies gain some independence. It is a hard pill to swallow, My Friends, but *so do we*. My observations—of the families I studied and of our own parenting community—convinced me we human parents tend to hibernate, too. As my children and their friends became adolescents, I detected something strange: parents who once hovered and helicoptered became much less attentive as the kids got older.

We check out during the teen years, in a variety of ways and for a variety of reasons. Sometimes our children and their behaviors scare us; we bury our heads in the sand ostrich-style because the truth is too tough to handle. Sometimes dealing with teenagers—and trying to maintain a sense of family harmony—becomes more painful than it's worth and we let them retreat to themselves so we can have some peace. Sometimes we conflate our own adolescent miseries with theirs and indulge their attempts to be popular or successful, ignoring their reprehensible actions and giving in to them when they don't deserve it. Most of the time, parents tend to hibernate because we're just dog-tired. It's understandable. Raising a family is exhausting.

When puberty knocks the family off course, some parents overcorrect by trying to gain control. It's a natural, kneejerk response for many of us; we try to right the ship by exerting power over our kids, their schedules and their transgressions. Some of us overcorrect the other way; when we feel overwhelmed, we check out. We relinquish control with a defeated shrug and adopt a hands-off stance toward our offspring. Both approaches—in opposite ways—abandon our teenagers. We abandon them when we don't trust them enough to make their own decisions but also when we leave them to make decisions for themselves before they're ready.

. . . .

PARENTING CASE STUDY:
How Hibernation Begins

I met Josie at the playground when our boys were in preschool. The kids bonded over shared superhero passions while Josie and I became lasting friends despite our epic differences. Josie was a fastidious housekeeper, a hyper organized family manager and (her words) "a ball of anxiety" especially when it came to her only child, the brilliant and affable Sebastion. Our home life, on the other hand, was messy, chaotic and laissez-faire. Although Josie brought her son over for endless playdates, I think she hosed him down with sanitizer every time they left. The Filholms had this effect on many of our friends; ours was a fun and loving house-hold but it made more traditional families a little nervous. In our rather dilapidated backyard, children worked on craft and science projects, practiced their skills in the batting cage, built structures with real tools and found objects, and painted themselves blue. It was also the loudest house in the 'hood due to a rotating band of young rock musicians in the basement. We kept our kids up too late and answered their questions about the birds and the bees with perhaps too much candor. Make no mistake, we had plenty of structure and our own strict boundaries (we were militant about table manners, good language and schoolwork and we—gasp!—permitted no video games in our house, ever) but to many in our circle, we seemed like feral parents.

I know Josie gagged when my three-year-old son licked play-ground rocks; I just shrugged. I think she prayed for my soul when I forgot to attend my first grader's Thanksgiving pageant and when

I opted for the slacker version of supporting teacher-appreciation breakfasts (two cases of bottled water instead of a handmade quiche). She herself was convinced Sebastian had been colicky as an infant because of her overwhelming pregnancy anxieties; I once saw her suffer palpitations when her son *almost* walked through some broken glass at the swimming pool. Whereas I gave my children full access to the library so long as they were reading, Josie vetted every book Sebastian checked out for content that might frighten, alarm or corrupt him. Speaking of libraries, Josie was the most rabid consumer of parenting literature I've ever known. Her habit of devouring every written word about vaccinations, behavior theories and online predators only fueled her nervousness but Josie was, to say the least, a vigilant parent when Sebastian was small.

I noticed a change when our boys were in early middle school. My sons came home from sleepovers at Josie's house newly excited about a very R-rated movie they'd watched and a notoriously violent video game they'd played. I wasn't offended, but surprised, that this exposure to questionable media had happened under Josie's roof. The plot thickened as Josie—and other friends previously known to be way more strict than the Filholm Family—agreed to a boy-girl sleepover for the eighth grade class (thanks to my own wayward adolescence, the very thought sent me into fits of distress). Meanwhile, I started to notice social media posts by our sons and some of their friends containing all manner of adolescent delight: bullying, drinking and drug use, selfies worthy of the Kardashian sisters. The other parents seemed strangely unmoved by all of it. Keep in mind, I was busy gathering research in the halls of an actual high school, so I knew enough to be freaked out when my young teenagers asked to go to "an all-night rave for high school kids at this dance club downtown." The fact that the proprietors of this lovely event "don't serve alcohol" comforted me not at all. I had specific knowledge of exactly what fuels the all-night rave culture; alcohol was the least of my concerns. But while I was giving my hard "no," our friends were dropping their kids off at the club with Uber fare and instructions to get home by 2:30 in the morning.

At this point in our parenting saga, my husband and I looked at each other and said, "What is going on here?" When, we wondered, had we turned into the prude and paranoid parents? Why do the same friends who once worried so aggressively about their younger kids suddenly seem to have so little concern about their vulnerable teenagers? Is everyone asleep on the job?

In search of answers, I turned to my living laboratory, the high school classroom. As I contemplated the possibility that parents turn a blind eye to the transgressions of our teenagers, I had the unique (and sometimes unfortunate) perspective of knowing the gritty reality of adolescent existence. Remember, I earned my PhD in Keepin' It Real during my time in the teaching trenches. Working with my students and their parents—and later, interviewing them for this book—illuminated some patterns of family behaviors. Many of us do check out when our children become adolescents. Before I start begging you not to hibernate (because our vulnerable teens need vigilant parents), let's think a bit about just why we feel so tempted to take a nap.

IT'S UNDERSTANDABLE: WE ARE EXHAUSTED.

Perhaps in direct proportion to how much we fretted and hovered while our children were young, parents are weary by the time puberty arrives. We are exhausted first of all because we have started to resent the neediness of our progeny, who by now seem pretty capable of cleaning up after themselves. We start to see how our efforts thus far (helping them learn to toilet, bathe, dress themselves and do basic household chores) might ease our daily burden and it's annoying when they don't pitch in. Willing help with the cooking and cleaning would be amazing but I'm not unreasonable; many days I would settle for a kitchen counter free of jock straps. Furthermore, even parents of tidy children are depleted by the time their eldest turns 11 or 12. Seriously, y'all. We deserve a medal for maneuvering the family through a single month of May (the annual perfect storm of recitals, tournaments, ceremonies, final projects and graduation parties. I call it Mayhem). Dear God. A fourth-grade science fair can drain the life right out of your veins. I don't know how parents of Girl Scouts survive cookie season without medication. If you have, in fact, engineered even one week-long camping trip for your nearest and dearest, you have the right to a spa vacation or a nervous break-down (your choice). Parents are burned out well before the teen years commence.

By the time our children demonstrate high-level skills like using fabric softener and maybe even changing a tire, well, we're ready to let our little cubs fend for themselves. Our teenagers encourage our hibernation as they practice wicked strategies to convince us they don't need us anymore. It is tempting to believe them when we're so tired and struggling so hard to get some semblance of our groove back. And they are just so *mean* to us! But parents must not hibernate. Our teenagers need us. They are worth saving. We cannot fall asleep on the job.

WE DON'T KNOW WHAT THE HECK WE'RE DOING.

Not only does Mama Bear hibernate when the going gets tough, she's got a lousy attitude for someone who lives amongst pubescent people. Thanks to her animal instincts, Mama Bear just seems so darned *sure* of herself. In my experience—and according to the hundreds of parents

I have studied—one thing is certain: when teenagers live in your home you rarely (if ever) feel confident or coolheaded. Even when things seem pretty good and the family is mostly getting along, it's a messy, muddled mind trip. Mama Bear never second-guesses herself, feels guilty or shows any signs of ambivalence. This attitude is supremely unhelpful for parents of teenagers. We spend most of our days feeling rotten at our jobs and unprepared for everything.

It is difficult to know how to parent teenagers because our job description is ambiguous from the moment of conception and almost guaranteed to inspire feelings of helplessness and inadequacy. Even within our own families, adults don't agree about the details of the work at hand. When kids hit puberty, the job itself gets more difficult (and often less enjoyable) thanks to their ever-changing, mind-bending demands. Meanwhile, as parents enter middle age we are especially vulnerable ourselves. We are spent from what feels like a marathon of parenting thus far and when our offspring get truculent, we take it personally. Our work is further complicated by that uncanny adolescent ability to find a parent's deepest wound and rub salt into it with germ-covered, teenaged fingers. We parent people who don't want to be parented. We love people who reject our love. Ours is a job of contradiction and hurt feelings and it's nearly impossible to define. Parents of teenagers, unlike old Mama Bear, rarely feel sure of themselves. It is unbelievably tempting to give up, check out, go to sleep on the job.

Everything we know about parenting evaporates when kids get hormonal, because 13-year-olds don't respond to anything the same way they did when they were six or seven. Gone are the days of feeling confident, protecting our children with atavistic aplomb, only to sink into our pillows each night exhausted but sure of our role in the world. With younger children, rules are clear and pretty simple to enforce. Stove, hot! Street, dangerous! Dipping your cookie in the toilet? Not the best choice! We know what young children need to learn and they are interested in all of it: the alphabet, numbers, the names of things, how trees grow and why it rains and how to play the piano and clean up your mess and tie your shoes and use the toilet and tell a joke and eat with a fork. Once they become teenagers, things are more complicated. The rules are difficult to negotiate amidst brave new technology and old-school adolescent rebellion. Teenagers—because it is their job—tell elaborate lies, crawl out windows, test limits, and beg us in many other ways to question values we hold dear.

Parents of teenagers need new role models because raising a family is difficult and awful by design. Nurturing people who can eventually survive on their own, contribute to society and enjoy their adult lives is an ugly, painful process. If we expect to know what we are doing—if we think we should feel sure of ourselves while raising teenagers—it's a million times harder. We need to cut ourselves some slack. Expecting perfection, certainty, family harmony or knowing what the hell we are doing eventually exhausts us; all we want to do is cover our eyes and hibernate.

. . . .

PARENTING CASE STUDY:
"It's Harder Than I Thought It Would Be"

Carl is one of the most successful people we know by almost any measure. He is a strong, strapping man, professionally accomplished, financially sound, a devoted father and loving husband: brilliant, funny, imposing, able, wise. We've known him and his family since those blissful early days of parenthood. On a recent summer evening I casually asked how things were going now that we all have adolescents in our homes. The light in Carl's eyes seemed to dim. He slumped a bit and suddenly looked older than his years. He sighed from deep within and said, "It's harder than I thought it would be." To all the world his two daughters are active, animated, polite young women. They are curious and engaged; they do well in

18

school. And yet I saw before me a man defeated. Something about daily family life was threatening to break his spirit. And I thought, if living with adolescents can cause a man like Carl to crumble, why should the rest of us expect anything different?

. . . .

BUT IT'S ALL PERFECTLY NORMAL.

Few parents of teenagers escape unscathed. Living with adolescents brings the best of us to our knees and it's easy to feel like a giant parenting failure most of the time. When our lovely children turn into angry malcontents, things tend to come apart at the seams: families, marriages, healthy self-identities. If you find yourself engaging in elaborate fantasies—like running away to join the circus, a monastery or a magical place where there is no laundry on the floor and no emails about missing homework— you are not alone.

Lately I've been pondering the first lines of Leo Tolstoy's *Anna Karenina*: "All happy families are alike; each unhappy family is unhappy in its own way." Maybe it's true. Maybe we are unique and set apart from one another by our struggles and strife. But these days, I doubt it. I gotta take issue with old Leo, now that I'm part of my own struggling family. Perhaps the details of each family's challenges are unique, but in the grand scheme of things, raising a family is hard for everyone. Most of the time, I feel like my crazy family is messed up in ways no one else will understand. And that's depressing, y'all. It's comforting to be reminded how perfectly normal it is to struggle when your kids are of a certain age. It happens to all of us. In this book I encourage all of us to take a new point of view: if we gain a better perspective of why it's so difficult to raise teenagers, we can focus on the light at the end of the tunnel. If we observe the normal (but nutty) patterns of family life, we can lean on each other and see our way to more peace and less strife.

AND OUR TEENAGERS NEED US.

It's hard to step back and gain this perspective because raising teenagers is bewildering and personal and painful (and exhausting). It's easy to sink into patterns of anger and chaos and it's easy for parents to lose sight of our purpose. When we do—when we fall asleep on the job of parenting our still growing children—we leave them awfully vulnerable. I am going to try and convince you that during the adolescent years, parents need to wake up. We need to look beyond Mama Bear and find ourselves some new role models, because on the rocky journey toward adulthood, our teenagers need parents and other adults to guide them. It is tempting to take their abuse personally and give up on them, to think, "they don't need me." I promise you, they do. Teenagers are hard-wired to reject some of the very things they crave, such as boundaries (and us). They will go to great lengths to convince you they don't need you, your rules, your opinions, your care or your concern. An adolescent will talk out of both sides of her mouth and often, his right hand literally does not know what his left hand is doing. But (as I will remind you again and again) they do need their parents. They need us differently than when they were learning to dress themselves but their needs are vast. Parents can take advantage of teenaged reality to help them grow into responsible adulthood. We have to dig deep and figure out how to meet their new (and ever-changing and confusing and frustrating) needs, but I repeat: they need us.

There is too much at stake for parents to hibernate. Teenagers are whirl-winds of angst, self-loathing and pretense who contradict themselves with wild passion. They can't help it. They are developmentally prone to behave recklessly, make awful decisions, test boundaries and act like little criminals. In many ways middle and high school kids need us more than they did when they were in third or fourth grades. They are almost adults, smack in the midst of actualizing their unique personalities. They need our help. When we lose our objectivity and let them hurt our feelings, we sometimes act more like wounded adolescents ourselves and less like helpful adults. When we leave them to themselves because they're so unpleasant to be around—or conversely, when we smother and save them because we don't trust them to gain their independence—we make their journeys more difficult.

And so, Dear Reader, in spite of our exhaustion, in spite of the Herculean task before us, I recommend we let Mama Bear go as a role model because hibernation will not serve us well during these difficult times.

WE LIVE IN HOPE.

If you—like Carl, like all of us—are feeling defeated by it all, I hope you'll keep reading. I hope you'll be convinced your kids are worth staying engaged for a few more years. I'll tell you why it's worth it (for them and for you) and I'll give you some practical ways to find your balance in the three-ring adolescent circus. My observations have taught me parents do best to know, protect and honor their adolescent children. There is not one new role model for the likes of us; there are many. In order to meet the demands of raising our children to adulthood, parents must find a balance, walk a fine line and quick-change between many, many hats. It's arduous work but—I promise!—our teenagers and our sanity are worth it in the long run.

In this book, we'll take a candid look at what's going on in a typical teenager's brain and body. As we explore some of the many ways teenagers upset the family (and why), I hope you'll recognize yourself and feel less alone. I hope you'll feel the comfort of knowing how normal and necessary the process is, no matter how impossible it seems sometimes. I will remind you often to check your balance on the high wire of raising a family. I will remind you how frequently we must make split decisions and practice superhuman discernment. I will remind you to stay vigilant.

I will remind you to laugh. When we work hard to know, protect and honor our teenagers, we can help pave their way to becoming the very best versions of themselves. I'll give you some tools—and some new role models—who can help us all.

Ten Things Your Family Might Ask When You Are Busy

I'm not saying this actually happened to me. I'm not saying it didn't. I'm just saying, if ever you have carved quiet time away to focus on a project (say, a fundraiser for your kids' school or tracking down that funny charge on your debit card), your family might interrupt and ask you these things. I'm just saying.

1. Do you know where the shop-vac is?
2. Does this chicken smell okay?
3. Can I take these flowers (just purchased and arranged in vase) to my girlfriend tomorrow? [Also, questions 3a and b: Do you have a different, smaller vase I could use? And could you show me where it is in the basement?]
4. Have you seen the checkbook?
5. Can you reschedule my orthodontist appointment?
6. Can I go to New York on a school trip in March (commitment money due Monday)?
7. Does this look like a rash or a bruise?
8. Could you please write "Will you go to Homecoming with me" in Russian cursive on this card?
9. Can you make my brother stop de-pantsing me in gym class?
10. Do you want a fajita (it was my understanding that the meal we ate two hours ago would serve as dinner)?

Let me be clear: I am privileged to be wife and mother to my family. I don't really mind answering any of these questions or performing any of these services. I am honored, in fact, to do so. It's just a tiny reminder of why this job of ours is kind of insane. When we sit down and try to focus, the interruptions are many, varied, and unpredictable. So it goes with parenting. It is so seldom convenient. It so rarely goes as planned. We are almost never truly prepared, for anything. It's tempting to hibernate and it's difficult to stay vigilant. Hang in there; stay the course; acknowledge the struggle. Our children are worth it in the end. And you might get to practice your high school Russian.

Chapter Two

How to Survive the Balancing Act: KNOW-PROTECT-HONOR

Running into a pole is a drag.
But never being allowed to run into a pole is a disaster.
~Daniel Kish, President, World Access for the Blind

DESPITE OUR EXPERIENCE, wisdom, and general aptitude for, you know, Life, raising adolescents can feel like showing up to a five-alarm fire with a squirt gun. Here's the good news: I've got some tools to help us feel a little more equipped for the challenge. I have observed parents—and their children—get through the funhouse of adolescence intact. After teaching hundreds of students and interviewing dozens of parents and teens, I realized the most effective parents share three general traits. The first is open eyes: the ability to step back from the chaos and evaluate every circumstance for what it is. These parents get to KNOW their kids. The second is strong arms: the willingness to step in and save their kids from harm if and when the situation demands, even if it's inconvenient or unpleasant. They PROTECT their teenagers from real and present danger. The third trait the parents I admire share is full hearts: the practical—but holy—knowledge that the process of growing up is hard but worth it. They HONOR and forgive their kids' unique, sometimes difficult, different than their own, journeys. I've condensed all their wisdom into:

The Three Most Important Questions to Ask While Raising Teenagers

1. Do I KNOW what's going on with my kid?
2. Must I step in to PROTECT my child from real and present danger?
3. Can I HONOR my child's unique journey toward adulthood?

KNOW-PROTECT-HONOR: this has become my shorthand. My mantra. My quick reminder of how to proceed when I get stuck in the rut of living with overgrown toddlers. When we can remember to step back, breathe, and ask ourselves these questions, parents find our way to more family harmony and less adolescent drama.

Whether they do so consciously or not, the parents I admire KNOW their kids' friends, their behaviors, their patterns, and enough about their secrets to keep the kids safe. They do not meddle or sweat the small stuff, but they maintain strict boundaries in order to PROTECT kids from some very real predators. These parents HONOR their teenagers. They forgive kids for being imperfect and in progress; they laugh at their foibles; they guide teenagers toward becoming the very best versions of themselves.

I will discuss these ideas—and how I arrived at them—in much greater detail. For now, try stepping back yourself when things spiral out of control with your teenager. Try it today! Try weighing each situation with clarity and candor. Ask yourself three things: "Do I KNOW what's really going on? Is there danger here from which I must PROTECT my child? Can I put my own needs, fears or feelings aside in order to HONOR the human being before me?" See if you gain any new insight. See if the conflict subsides, even just a bit. But stay vigilant! I'll give you a whole crew of new role models beyond Mama Bear who will help us KNOW, PROTECT and HONOR our teenagers (and ourselves). Meanwhile, keep reading for more on why this job of raising teenagers is so tough (it really is) and how to make sense of it (you can do it)!

PARENTING CASE STUDY:
The Half-Second Test

My favorite episode of *Invisibilia*, an NPR podcast by Lulu Miller and Alix Spiegel, investigates human and societal expectations through eyesight, or lack of it (2015). Daniel Kish is a blind man who taught himself from a very early age to navigate his world with a series of clicks of his tongue. Now an expert in human echolocation and founder/president of World Access for the Blind, he trains young blind people to use the echolocation system. In the moment I love best, we listen to a five-year-old child, his godmother, and Mr. Kish working on the boy's developing skills. They approach a busy highway. The young boy uses his cane and a series of clicks to determine where he is. As he gets dangerously close to oncoming traffic, his godmother steps in and pulls him back. Mr. Kish grimaces, disappointed. He insists children—especially those with limited sight—need to do things for themselves or be rendered helpless. He knows it's tough to extend independence; most sighted people will jump in a "half-second too soon and rob the blind student of a learning moment." He believes that moment of challenge, even danger, is a place of growth. The kid's godmother understands the danger of rescuing him a half-second too early—he needs to learn how to make that judgment call—but "at the end of the day she is far more concerned about the half-second too late."

So much of parenting feels this way; a half-second too early, we rob our kids of the chance to grow and learn. A half-second too late and we lose them to the dangers of the world. It's a constant balancing act. Parents of teenagers make a million decisions. We face situations and hear ourselves uttering phrases we could not fathom when our families were young and fresh. We are required to do contrary, confusing things when adolescents live in our homes. Sometimes it's best to make teenagers stick to their commitments and finish what they've started. Other times, a child is best served by quitting (a class or activity or friend or hobby). Every situation is different. Every child is different. What works with one kid fails with the next; what worked in the past stops working.

Sometimes we have to leap into action with the muscle and swiftness of a cheetah. At other times we have to sit with the silent patience of a monk. When we're faced with mercurial adolescent people, parents may be called upon to act hard as nails one day, gentle as lambs the next. As I studied parents and teenagers I took notes on what seemed to be most effective when family life spins out of control. I learned, as I have discussed, that parents of teens tend to hibernate—to disengage, to turn a blind eye to their kids—because maintaining this balancing act is exhausting. I also noticed what happens when parents stay vigilant instead. No matter what their families look like, regardless of their specific parenting challenges, the parents who seem to survive the storm (and whose kids thrive, too) tend to KNOW, PROTECT and HONOR their adolescent children.

Raising teenagers is a series of micro moments designed to flummox us. Every struggle is unique: every child, every situation, every frustrating challenge springs like a leak in the hull of our family ship. Every day— often many times in a day—living with teenagers requires us to make split-second, adult decisions. It is exhausting and it's tempting to look the other way or take a nap or check out entirely. The parents I admire most do the opposite. When teenaged drama threatens their peaceful course, these parents treat it like a wake-up call.

This vulnerable, chaotic time in our family lives feels like a three-ring circus and we seek the precarious balance of a tightrope walker. We try to find the fine line that gives our teenagers freedom within boundaries, space to make mistakes and learn, permission to find autonomy and develop their own personalities. Also, we want to keep them safe. How do we find this middle ground between over- and under-parenting? What does the elusive balance look like, between authoritarian and permissive parenting? [1]

I think the ultimate parent—a model for myself and all of us—looks much like our tightrope walker, who stays stay poised amidst the *sturm und drang*, who remains steady while the calliope plays and the lions roar and the clowns come endlessly out of tiny cars. Parents who raise responsible, well-adjusted children stay alert, centered and detached from the melee. Parents, like tightrope walkers, might lean a little too far in one direction when adolescence throws us off our balance. To stay upright, we must recognize the error, lean the other way and keep walking. When teenagers threaten that balance, we can try to remain flexible, ready to pivot and adjust. We can expect to be challenged and we can be prepared to respond appropriately. We can anticipate trouble ahead and make adjustments to our routines. And before making any decisions at all regarding our hormonal, dramatic, sensitive, adolescent daughters and sons, we can ask three vital questions: Do I KNOW? Must I PROTECT? Can I HONOR?

Because it's a visual world, I've turned the whole sequence into the flow chart on the next page. Each of our new role models will serve us in a specific way. The task of parenting is too complex and complicated for us to seek one new role model. We need many as we respond appropriately to the unpredictable needs of our teenagers.

29

HOW TO TAKE A PARENTING TIME-OUT

Step back from every complicated situation and

ASK:

Do I **KNOW** what's really going on with my teens?

YES . . . . **NO**

watch them like a FALCON	study them like a PRIVATE INVESTIGATOR	ambush them like a NINJA

. . . .

then **ASK:**

Must I **PROTECT** my teens from any real danger?

YES . . . . **NO**

guard them like a SOLDIER	work them like a PERSONAL TRAINER	rest them like a PRESCHOOL TEACHER

. . . .

then **ASK:**

Can I **HONOR** the unique (not mine!) journey of my teens?

YES . . . .

guide them like a MENTOR	forgive them like an ARTIST	push them like a FALCON

. . . .

THEN, AND ONLY THEN:

decide your course of action (or inaction).

PARENTING CASE STUDY:
Surf's Up! (Know-Protect-Honor in Action)

Watching great parents in action gives me a little thrill. They do it effortlessly. In the heat of the moment, in public, in any circumstance at all, great parents know, protect and honor their children. One of my favorite Great Parenting Moments happened when the father in question was waist deep in the Pacific Ocean. Our friend Chris, a local Maui boy, was teaching our mainland sons how to surf. Meanwhile, his seven-year-old daughter Kiele paddled around the gentle waves, practicing on her own board. After half an hour on the water, Kiele had floated far enough away to panic us landlubbers. Her daddy, however, kept calm.

KNOW

Chris knew exactly where his daughter was without training his eyes on her constantly. An island native himself raising three Hawai'ian girls, he knows Kiele's strength as well as the conditions of the water. Chris also knew the currents at this particular beach; even if his daughter drifted away helplessly, she would eventually float around a lava outcropping into a shallow eddy on the other side.

PROTECT

Kiele is an experienced spear fisher who accompanies her daddy on increasingly challenging dives, but Chris doesn't take her out in really rough water. He has taught her to respect the inherent dangers of the ocean and keep safety in mind; he has given her the skills and tools to save herself in crisis. Chris challenges his adventurous daughter within the limits of her age, size and ability. The ocean that day seemed wild and dangerous to us, but to Chris and Kiele, it was like a stroll through a neighborhood park.

HONOR

As we stood worried on the shore, as Kiele drifted ever further from our party, Chris calmly turned to his little girl and called, "dig deep!" It was a champion moment of parenting. Within the boundaries of knowing and protecting her, he honored his daughter's ability to figure it out for herself. "Dig deep" reminded Kiele to use her many resources to get out of a tough situation. And she did.

I suspect this girl will be able to do exactly the same in later years, when teenagers find themselves in different kinds of tough situations. Don't we all long for our teenagers to "dig deep," call upon their inner strength, and paddle away from all kinds of danger?

(In this case, names have not been changed. Good parenting comes with few daily rewards; Chris should hear the shout-out. Credit is due, too, to his lovely wife Aki, who is fierce in her own million ways.)

Chapter Three

It's Only Teenage Wasteland:
Who Left the Demon in the Bed?

O that it could be proved
That some night-tripping fairy had exchanged
In cradle-clothes our children where they lay . . .
~Henry IV, Part I

PARENTING CASE STUDY:
What Happened to My Kid?

Under the florescent lights of the school gym, Nancy's eyes welled with tears. In a voice touched with panic and sadness she asked me, "Is he going to be okay?" Her son Ben—normally an academic superstar—was carrying a solid 'D' in my freshman English class and hadn't turned in a scrap of homework for six weeks. Worse yet, she said, he had become sullen and secretive. His usual gregarious personality and passion for joke telling had morphed into bitterness, sarcasm and refusal to make conversation with anyone— even family and friends he had recently adored. He had become mean, she explained as she choked back her sobs, especially to his parents and siblings, which was making everyone miserable. Ben's insults had become so nasty and so personal it was hard to ignore him and act like everything was okay.

Ben had been a motivated, champion swimmer since he was quite young. His passion—along with his training and competition—had shaped the family's schedule for years. Now, suddenly, Ben seemed to resent both the sport and his parents' support. He was verbally abusive when they got him up for morning practice and refused to keep track of his own equipment. When Nancy scolded him for another missing pair of trunks or goggles, Ben would threaten to quit swimming forever and swear he hated it, anyway. As a matter of fact, she admitted, a couple of weeks ago Ben had skipped out on afternoon workout to hang out in a nearby park. He lied about it to his parents—which angered them—but his response upon getting caught absolutely flummoxed them. Pressed to explain his actions, Ben just shrugged his shoulders and mumbled. Part of the trouble, Nancy surmised, was his new group of friends. Ben seemed to have dropped all the buddies he'd grown up with— good kids whom his parents knew and loved—in favor of some awfully sketchy characters.

Nancy's hardworking son had turned lazy. The boy once so passionate about so many pursuits—model rockets, growing tomatoes, reading Harry Potter—had become apathetic about every single thing under the sun. The social child with the engaging personality had isolated himself from the world. "He would be plugged into his headphones 24 hours a day if we let him," Nancy cried. "I just don't know what happened. It's like my son is gone." She asked again, "Is he going to be okay?"

changeling ˈtʃeɪndʒlɪŋ

1. a child surreptitiously or unintentionally substituted for another.

2. (in folklore) an ugly, stupid, or strange child left by faeries in place of a pretty, charming child.

If you have adolescent children, Nancy's lament at a parent-teacher conference might sound familiar. Whether you feel like you are losing your family, your hair, your tenuous grip on reality, or your ever-loving mind, once kids hit puberty your life gets jacked up, and fast. Hang in there, moms and dads . . . you're not alone. We should talk about it over a glass of wine. As soon as possible. Preferably someplace public, away from sharp objects, and filled with reasonable, peaceful people over the age of 30. Who will bring us more wine. I mean it. Let's make a date.

If, on the other hand, your kids are younger—say, under the age of 10 or 11—listen up. If they still generally like you and smell pretty good most of the time, drop this book right now and go smell them. I mean it—put your nose as far into their personal spaces as they will allow and inhale the sweet aroma of them. If they will still let you smother them with kisses, do that too. Do it while you still can, My Friend, because soon all that is going to change. (Once you have finished your smelling and kissing, please return to this book. It all turns in the blink of an eye and you might as well start preparing. But hang on tight. What you are about to hear may make your head spin. In this case, smell again. Kiss again. Repeat.)

Medieval literature is rife with tales of the swapped child, or changeling: a troll or faerie switched with a human child under the cloak of nighttime. It's a haunting theme; parents find hideous, malformed beasts in place of their cherubic, beautiful children. Scholars tell us the trope helped people justify unexplained diseases and disorders. Anyone who has spent time with teenagers knows it is also the only explanation for what happens when our kids hit puberty. Sweet and loving daughters and sons are replaced—it seems like it happens overnight—by unrecognizable creatures.

That's the worst part: it sneaks up on you. There is no formal announcement: "Mom, Dad, I've made my transition into adolescence! Things are about to get bananas." Puberty comes upon you like a thief in the night, and there is little you can do to prepare yourself. If you are at all like me, you knew the adolescent years would be tough. You knew it because you were once a teenager yourself. You may, in fact, have uttered words to this effect: "Dear God, I hope my kid doesn't act like me . . . ." Maybe you heard the parents' curse: "I hope someday you have a kid of your own who acts just like you . . . ." You have read parenting books, attended seminars, baked millions of cupcakes and stayed involved in their schools. You secretly pat yourself on the back about how well your kids are turning out and what a great job you are doing not repeating the mistakes your parents made. You are prepared for—almost looking forward to—the kooky teen antics which will challenge your family someday, because you know you've got this.

Oh, Dear Reader. Brace yourself. It may take you by surprise . . . and it is ugly.

> Going right through try to stay cool,
> Going through, staying cool . . .
> As we get older and stop making sense . . .
> (Stop making sense, making sense)
> **~Talking Heads**

DO YOU HAVE AN ADOLESCENT ON YOUR HANDS?

As early as age 10, kids begin cultivating habits and attitudes which blossom into full-fledged adolescence. It can be a shock because suddenly everything stops making sense. Poor Nancy at that parent-teacher conference thought her son was gone for good. Because the changes in his personality seemed so sudden, aggressive and frightening, she assumed he had turned into a different person. She thought these new behaviors and attitudes were signs of his burgeoning (and awful) adult personality. Of course this wasn't true. Veteran teachers are the perfect people to ask, "Is my kid going to be okay?" because they see it all—and they see it year after year. Best of all, they see freshmen grow into seniors and then college students and even grown-up professionals. Sometimes all a parent really needs to hear is, "this too will pass." Because a heck of a lot of the time, it does. Ben's behavior was indeed a phase—a function of hormones—and I am happy to report he turned out just fine! I eventually taught him senior English and he had grown right back into his engaging, funny, curious, motivated self.

There is no doubt teens require different parenting skills and tactics than they did when they were younger. The whole family needs to adjust to meet their changing needs and demands and abject craziness. They are difficult but they are vulnerable, and parents can do much to guide and protect them. The sooner we recognize signs of adolescent behavior, the sooner we can adjust and properly tend our new landscape. If we can name a thing, we can understand it. If we know what it is, we may be less afraid of it (and I'm here to tell you, teenagers can be pretty scary). Knowing the nature of the beast figures mightily in our ability to tame it. And so. If you've heard one or more of the following come out of your mouth lately, step back and take inventory. Is it possible you have an adolescent on your hands? (Take heart: your kids aren't rotten or ruined, at least not permanently. They're just entering the wasteland of adolescence.)

. . . .

Eight Things You Might Hear Yourself Say
If You Have an Adolescent on Your Hands:

1. "That's the fourth jacket you have lost this year!" (or phone, textbook, glasses, key, mouthguard or . . .). This is often where it begins.
2. "You have an F! An actual F!" If a perennial excellent pupil suddenly loses interest or ability when it comes to school, you're probably *in it.*
3. "But you love gymnastics! You can't just quit!" Likewise horses, baseball, groups of friends and other passions. Dropping things they have loved all their lives is a sure sign: you've got a teenager in your house.
4. "Can you say something positive for a change?" Gradually (but also suddenly) their negative commentary on the world will overwhelm you. When every sentence begins, "You know what sucks . . . " or "You know what's cheap about . . . " or "You know what I hate . . . ," you've entered Teenage Wasteland.
5. "Who ate all the cereal?" If your child eats like an animal and/ or sleeps like a rock, adolescence is right around the corner.
6. "What did you just say? I swear, I can't understand you!" Does the kid who spoke in full sentences before her second birthday now mumble, grunt and spit her replies to you? Check. That's a teenager.
7. "Please remove your headphones when I am speaking to you." The tendency to retreat from us into their own, surly little worlds? Particularly when that checking out is accompanied by an angry, private soundtrack? Yes, indeed: that's

adolescence! (7a: "Will you just come out of your bedroom for a change?")

8. "Why is the bathroom door locked?" A sudden (and suspicious) need for privacy is a telltale sign. Times, along with hormonal little bodies, they are a changin'.

· ·

Well, Dear Reader, where do you stand? If you recognize yourself or your child here, welcome to the wonderful, wild world of adolescence!

My friends (who are far more civilized than I am) beg me not to say this, but hanging out with a teenager can feel a lot like being a battered spouse. People balk at this analogy because they worry it minimizes or pokes fun at the very real and serious problem of domestic violence. I assure you, levity is not my intent. I use this model of dysfunction precisely because it is so grave and the patterns of abuse are so predictable and devastating. Here's what I have observed with both my students and my own kids: parents grow used to an icy distance between themselves and their teens. We learn to expect harsh criticism about our shoes, our living-room furniture, our ideas about life, the sound of our voices when we express such ideas. We seldom do anything right. Our presence—pretty much anywhere—might invoke humiliation or rage or both. Verbal insults in public become so commonplace we hardly notice anymore. And then, for some reason (we learn not to ask too many questions) our child treats us well. She says, "I love you, Mom." He says, "Thank you, Dad." He clears his own dishes or she remembers our birthday without being prompted. And then, like the battered spouse, we forgive and forget. We see a ray of hope in the darkness! We think, it hasn't been that bad! He loves me! She was nice to me! I can survive another day! And then the magic moment melts away, leaving the changeling who has replaced your child to continue dispensing that daily dose of nastiness.

Sounds similar to the patterns of an abusive relationship, no? Perhaps the analogy is too harsh, but either way, it's crazy-making. Living with—and trying to communicate with—adolescents is like being on a carnival ride that looks fun and innocent, but once you are strapped in for good, it hurls you so painfully through time and space you wonder if a sadistic clown is at the helm. The whole world looks confusing and scary when you're stuck on a joyride gone bad.

I am here to tell you they do mature. One of the great joys of teaching is having these very same troublemakers check back six or seven or eight years later to tell you all about their plans for grad school or the Peace Corps or a real-live paying job. In the meantime, it's good to know what we are up against.

Every teenager and every scenario demands a different response, a different new role model, a different perspective. Families are complex social systems in a constant state of change. By definition, we form interdependent bonds with our children and spouses. According to the natural demands of human development, these relationships evolve and change over and over again. While we live as a unit we perpetually redefine and redistribute our roles, expectations and relationships. Here's the thing: teenagers are like caterpillars who have gone into cocoon. They're in that unrecognizable, awkward, even ugly stage from which they will emerge transformed. They are changing so much they sort of don't resemble themselves from day to day. Eighteenth-century philosopher Jean-Jacques Rousseau (1762) described this metamorphosis as the second birth of a human being. The first, he said, is physical—born into existence—and the second is a birth of consciousness: born into life. It's challenging, serious stuff. When teenagers retreat to their bedrooms, tune into their headphones or hide behind offensive fashion choices, they are seeking a cocoon of protection and isolation where they can do the painful, awkward work of growing into their adult personalities.

The only thing truly predictable about teenagers is their unpredictability. When all is said and done it can be helpful to remember that the little punks are becoming butterflies. As tough as it can be, it's up to parents to find balance and provide some consistency because teenagers—by design—are fairly incapable of doing so for themselves. To underscore that point, let's take a good look at exactly what's going on in the hormonal brains of these adolescent people.

Chapter Four

They Act Their Age: The Open Window of the Teenage Brain

We are all faced with a series of opportunities—
brilliantly disguised as insoluble problems.
~John Gardner

WHAT IS ADOLESCENCE? LET'S DEFINE OUR TERMS.

Before we go much further it is probably wise to name the beast. I write about teenagers and adolescents pretty interchangeably but that's just for convenience. As you may be aware, our progeny often become unrecognizable well before the thirteenth birthday. You may also know (and if not, I'm sorry to be the harbinger of doom) how goofy they act well into their twenties. True story: the period marked by reckless behavior and questionable decision-making begins earlier than we might expect and lingers much longer than we might prefer. "Teenager" technically means a person between the ages of 13 and 19, of course, but the definition of "adolescent" depends upon both biology and culture. Experts agree about the onset of adolescence—it's puberty—but its ending is less clear. When sex hormones rev up the brain and body, a period of rapid growth and maturation begins adolescence. As the prefrontal cortex works to catch up with the explosive limbic system, human experience is marked by impulsivity and heightened emotion—all the trappings of "adolescence." Generally, the age of adolescence ends when physical maturation meets autonomy from the family of origin, whether that means marriage or other choices and experiences. In theory—if not always in practice—those who establish independence from the family unit are ready to start families of their own. Their penchant for reckless behavior has diminished. They can plan ahead and act according to long-term rewards and consequences. When these cognitive functions mature, adolescence ends and adulthood begins (Steinberg, 2014).

In all cultures and times throughout recorded human history, the mortality rate among boys spikes a few years after puberty. It's called "the accident hump" by sociologists and statisticians (Goldstein, 2011). A middle-school teacher I admire jokes about the "testosterone poisoning" responsible for so much seventh-grade-boy behavior. Turns out, it's a real thing. The universal spike in teenaged death is a direct result of the chemistry laboratory inside their skulls. Teenagers (especially males) are prone to recklessness and risk-taking. No doubt about it. Girls express their impulsivity in less overtly violent—but I am convinced just as damaging—ways.

As their ability to regulate themselves develops (and it does!) teenagers are hard at work solidifying their identities. The upside of their chaotic little brains is an intense period of growth and potential. The plasticity of their neural development means adolescents are shaped by outside influences, including parents, teachers and others who care about them. Dr. Lawrence Steinberg, in his 2014 exploration of the teenage brain *The Age of Opportunity*, explains that—thanks to environmental and genetic factors—puberty begins at an earlier age in every generation, while young adults are becoming autonomous at a collectively older age. Adolescence in America lasts longer than it ever has; the teen decade is only the middle part. I know the thought of a longer adolescence might cause panic, but we do best to see it as a great opportunity, indeed! It's an extended chance to have an influence on the lives and development of our not-quite-grown-up children.

As we examine a parent's (impossible) job description and the most important tasks of adolescence, I want you to feel less alone and less hopeless when your kids—whether they are 10 or 22—act their age. I hope to give you a new point of view and practical advice for how to survive these crazy-making years. By way of definition, then, I am writing about the human people whose bodies have started to mature beyond the scope of their reasoning and self-control. If I write "teenager" but your kid is only 12 (or if your kid is 24), I hope you'll forgive the inaccuracy. By "teenager," I mean "slightly unreasonable person prone to fits of unexpected emotion."

Ten Things Teenagers Cannot Do

If you're butting heads with someone in early adolescence, here's a developmental reminder: teenagers act their age. There are a few things you should keep in mind. Through no fault of their own, most people aged 12 to 15 in middle America simply cannot be expected to:

1. Focus on anything at all when an insect, spider or puppy is nearby.
2. Regain composure within two hours of anyone farting.
3. Sit in a chair 100% of the time without falling out of it (this mostly applies to boys, but it is true. Mark my words: your boys will fall out of their chairs).
4. Explain why completed homework has not been turned into the teacher (they truly do not know).
5. Follow instructions the first time they are given.
6. Understand their own bursts of anger, tears, or apathy.
7. Control their own volume (this mostly applies to girls, but it is true. Whether they are laughing, screaming or yelling, few things on the planet are louder than freshmen girls).
8. Tell the truth about their feelings (they don't understand them and they can't explain them and they feel victimized by them).
9. View themselves with candor and love (they see themselves through the eyes of their peers, the media, and who-knows-what other influences. It's very confusing).
10. Organize anything: their rooms, backpacks, even the sentences forming as they speak.

I know all this because teaching a class of freshmen feels like being trapped with a herd of knife-bearing three-year-olds. A vocabulary lesson can erupt into chaos if the teacher relaxes for even a moment. The best-laid plans of mice and men go oft awry, as Steinbeck reminds us in that perennial freshman English favorite. Teachers make lesson plans and students thwart them. Inventing creative, surprising, specific ways to torture us is well within a teenager's wheelhouse. It is impossible to prepare. There is no rule book. Spending time with teenagers is confusing, frustrating, humbling, and exhausting.

Teachers learn the hard way about lesson plans. Like any plans we have for our children, they do not exist in a vacuum. We teach actual, live human beings and it gets pretty messy. If we expect teenagers to play along and respect the rules of the game, we're doomed. As teachers and parents know (but I marvel at my perpetual need to be reminded), our children seldom play by the rules. Instead, they dress like hookers or draw penis graffiti on their notebooks. We have to formulate a new game plan when their hormones take over. On the bright side, living with teenagers keeps us in the moment. They are a constant invitation to remain flexible, keep learning, and see the world through new eyes. Meeting them where they are requires vigilance and superhuman tenacity but we know it's worth it. When we break through a sullen stare and connect with a teenager, when we get a glimpse of the funny, confident, fascinating grown-up lurking behind the angst (almost but not quite ready to see the light of day) we can see it's worth it. Staying on the sunny side of the street is easier said than done when we're faced with real-live hooligans, but it's worth it every single time.

BRAIN CHEMISTRY: EMOTIONS AND PLEASURE RULE.

Nothing in the life of an adolescent person seems in control. Their thoughts and emotions are tangled and often scary. They are astute enough to recognize hypocrisy but naive enough to be frightened by it. In fact, much is beyond their control. During adolescence, the human brain is developing and organizing itself for the demands of adult-hood. As soon as the puberty engines start revving, emotions rule the brain and body. It takes years for higher-level cognitive functions to catch up. Adolescence is a time of impulse, sensation, immediacy and growth. The body and brain explode with chemical and physical activity. Young people are super vulnerable to sensations and feelings because it's all limbic system and dopamine receptors during these years—whim and pleasure and thrillseeking. The prefrontal cortex—which controls impulse, weighs consequences and regulates action—lags behind in development. In short, they're slaves to their desires because everything good feels so much better to a teenager (Steinberg, 2014). Until that frontal lobe is fully formed, there's not much preventing kids from obeying the dictates of their pleasure sensors, all the time. We can't trust them to make sound decisions because—mind, body and spirit—they are wired to do the opposite.

SENSATIONS ARE EVERYTHING.

You know how certain smells or sounds from your youth can evoke specific memories? Personally, the aroma of Bonne Bell Bubblegum lip gloss, stale Coors Light or a Russian Olive tree in the month of May can send me into intense high school reverie of one sort or another. (Never mind the power of certain Grateful Dead, Steve Miller Band or Pink Floyd songs to transport me right back to my freshman dorm room.) We are all sensory sponges during those salad days; adolescents literally see colors more vividly, taste food more intensely and feel the wind on their faces more keenly than they will at any other time in their lives (Steinberg, 2014).

Even when they act exactly like they're not listening, teenagers are experiencing, feeling and absorbing everything around them. When I taught high school I took advantage of their condition by making my classroom beautiful and pleasant. I eschewed overhead fluorescent lights for lamps and strings of small bulbs. Whenever possible, I used solid wood furniture and played good music during passing periods. I treated the walls as thoughtfully as I do my own home and kept the room smelling sweet. For adolescent people (and all of us—but more so for them), good feelings beget more good feelings. I primed their brains to soak up as much grammar and literary analysis as possible by appealing to their hyper-reactive senses.

Now that my former students are all grown up, they remember me for many things. Sometimes, it's stuff I endeavored to teach them—how to write a solid argument or deconstruct a text—but other times it's the sensory experience we shared. They thank me for introducing them to reggae-rapper Matisyahu, for hanging butterflies from the ceiling, for offering a cozy respite from the high school storm. I did not always leave my students with the lessons I intended because they soak up *everything* during those sensitive years. But I left them with something. It's a good reminder of how important it is to tread lightly with impressionable teenagers.

THEIR BRAINS ARE OPEN WINDOWS.

Should we doubt just how impressionable they are, we need only look at recent research confirming the brain's intense "plasticity" during adolescence. The malleable nature of the brain allows teens to learn from experience and adapt to the environment. It is a quality that engenders more of the same: brains challenged and nourished during these years will develop into more resilient adult brains. The brain is primed to learn from new experiences during adolescence. Dr. Steinberg employs several useful analogies to help us understand this plasticity, which is heightened during the early years of childhood and again during adolescent development. Wet clay is reminiscent of our brains, he writes: easily shaped by outside experience when it is raw, nearly impossible to manipulate once it hardens. Electrical wiring, too, helps us understand: during times of greater plasticity, the brain makes and strengthens new, more efficient connections. Teenaged brains are hard at work rewiring, ensuring full power from all outlets in adulthood. The metaphor I love best is the open window of the brain. During adolescence, its malleable nature means the window is thrown wide open to the influences of the outside world (without the protection of a screen or shutters). Along with sweet summer breezes and bird songs, the open-window brain lets in pollution, vermin and weather. A plastic, moldable brain is an opportunity to experience the fullness of life. It is also a liability, susceptible to all the negative influences the world has to offer.

Here again is a reason not to check out, parents. (I know I sound like a broken record, but it's vital!) When our children are tiny we believe we have a big influence in their lives. Otherwise we wouldn't invest in all those Baby Einstein videos and mommy-and-me yoga classes. It can be a hard pill to swallow, but the teenaged brain is similarly receptive to our input and influence. If we engage, we can help our kids take advantage of their awesome new brains. They can actually learn to be better adults because these are the years when they are learning to self-regulate. They are learning the skills of making plans and following them, controlling their behavior, working with other people and understanding long-term consequences. When these tasks are interrupted, people tend to repeat mistakes and patterns of reckless behavior well into adulthood.

BE AWARE: OF THE DANGERS AND THE POSSIBILITIES.

The plasticity of the adolescent brain is a primary reason kids shouldn't use drugs during these years. There is a close association between exposure to drugs during puberty and adult addiction. In early adolescence—during puberty, especially—drugs like nicotine and alcohol (and worse) can permanently affect the brain. Regular use can do long-term damage and certainly it can activate a dangerous pattern of abuse. These substances mess with the reward system in the brain just as all that heavy rewiring is taking place. A teenager's high is more intense than an adult's, remember, because they're sensation sponges (everything feels more intense). That awesome intensity can also turn more quickly into dependence. As the brain forms, it gets used to relying on a foreign substance in order to experience even normal amounts of pleasure. A teenaged brain can quickly develop a need for the drug (or drink or chemical) in order to feel okay; it stops being about getting high and becomes about feeling normal. It is vital to respect their great susceptibility before the age of 15, but the brain remains in its super-malleable state into the twenties (Steinberg, 2014). I'll say it now and I'll say it again: under the age of 15 (approximately—why not just say 18 or 21 to be safe?), drugs and alcohol are terrible for the developing brain. The consequences are serious and often permanent. Kids shouldn't be messing around with that stuff and we should do everything we can to prevent access.

Adolescent brains are also super susceptible to other negative influences, such as stress and fatigue. It's our job (while they are growing) to protect them from truly damaging influences on their development. It's their job to rage against every boundary we set. They are predisposed to make reckless choices and we are tasked with keeping them safe. Holden Caulfield doesn't mention if the kids he's trying to save from running over that crazy cliff are simultaneously pelting him with rotten tomatoes and making his job impossible. Our teenagers are doing just that: trying to prevent us from doing our job of helping them. As always, it's tough to find the fine line between loving them and strangling them. One of the very best things we can do for our kids, though, is help them grow up with healthy, functioning brains.

Because the adolescent brain is young and malleable, parents have a shot at making a difference. The open window of adolescence means we can make an impression on our teenagers. I will beg you to look at the big picture, choose your battles, see the forest and ignore some of the trees. We cannot, of course, protect them from everything. Part of our job is preparing them to handle whatever the big, wide world has to offer, including negative influences and personal setbacks. We can't shelter them, even when we wish we could. As I will discuss in greater detail, I believe the best refuge we can give young adults is the shelter of really good brains that work well for the rest of their lives: brains that operate to full capacity, think critically, discern and synthesize and create. Most importantly, we can help them build brains that can self-regulate. If my kids grow up to be people who can delay gratification for later rewards and remain true to themselves despite external stimuli, I shall be quite pleased.

HOW PARENTS CAN HELP: SCAFFOLD THEIR ABILITIES.

How do teenagers learn to regulate themselves (their reactions, actions and choices) while their brains work against the process? By being regulated. We learn in baby steps. Educators talk of scaffolding: as students learn to master new skills, teachers (and parents) give successive levels of support, then remove the structures as they are no longer needed. Learning to ride a bicycle is a great example. We wouldn't expect a toddler to ride a full-sized cruiser. Maybe we start our kid on a balance bike or a tricycle. Perhaps we equip their first big-kid bicycle with training wheels for a time. Maybe we hold the back of the seat and run behind, until at some point we let go and watch our kid ride down the block all alone.

We provide scaffolding to support them while they learn; when they are ready for independence we let them complete tasks on their own.

Recently an almost-three-year-old reminded me how naturally we scaffold life lessons for toddlers. We were heading out for a day of fun and I asked her to put on her shoes while I grabbed my things. At first, she railed against the very idea and cried, "I caaaaan't! I can't do it! I don't know how!" In the moment she really couldn't put on her own shoes. She was frustrated and maybe even frightened by the task itself and she lacked the tools to get the job done. Because three-year-old tantrums are easily shaken off, I remained calm and endeavored to teach her. I sat with her on the floor and we examined her shoes. We talked about how much easier they are to slip onto feet when the straps are open. We experimented with a few approaches to putting them on. We discovered the task was best accomplished by placing the toes of the shoes against a wall, slipping the feet in one at a time, and closing the strap with a hearty, "pull, push, snap!" We practiced the routine several times. Of course she could put on her shoes! And of course she was proud from that moment on to tell anyone who would listen all about her new "big-girl" skill. We do it naturally with little kids: we scaffold life lessons for them.

Teenaged tantrums are so much uglier, it can be difficult to remain calm when they need guidance. The scaffolding they require—the life skills adolescents need to practice—are more complicated. I believe the most important skill to scaffold for teens is the ability to think critically about risk, reward and long-term consequences. If they can regulate themselves as adults, they have a chance at making the most of their amazing brains. But self-regulation is a skill they cannot master for themselves (yet). We need to get down on the floor with them (figuratively speaking) and help them practice these strange new tasks. In the meantime, it's our job to protect their developing, open-window brains.

INVINCIBILITY: IT'S NOT JUST AN ADOLESCENT THING.

If parents think as carefully about the stimuli we provide our teenagers as we did when they were babes in our arms, we can help protect them from the world and from themselves. We can stack the deck in their favor. We can make it more difficult for them to do really dangerous things when they feel reckless. Believe it or not, teenagers basically understand the consequences of unprotected sex, drinking, smoking and not completing their homework. They just don't think the consequences apply to them. Before we write off their confidence as another function of adolescence, consider this: when it comes to our health, people of all ages make choices we know are bad for us. Adults—like it or not—really do ask kids to "do as I say, not as I do." Sure, teenagers feel invincible, but don't we all? Our bad adult habits prove we feel invulnerable most of our lives. Even if their parents are models of personal health, think of the contradictory messages kids receive from the adult world. Think about advertising from their point of view: a lot of things that are bad for us sure seem glamorous, everywhere we look. Adults seem hypocritical to teenagers and often we are. The difference between them and us, however, is that crazy, plastic, post-pubescent brain. They have too much to lose while their brains are still developing. It's a matter of protecting them even when our rules for them are contrary to our own behavior.

Chapter Five

Teenagers Are the New Toddlers: Except They're Not Actually Toddlers

She's got eyes of the bluest skies
As if they thought of rain
I hate to look into those eyes
And see an ounce of pain
~Guns N' Roses, *Sweet Child of Mine*

I INVITE ALL parents at this stage to breathe deeply and imagine our children as they were when they were toddlers. There is much written about the "U-shaped" demands of parenting; it's tough when the kids are little, then it gets relatively easier, then it gets nuts again when they turn on us after puberty. I want to convince you how very similar teenagers are to their toddler selves, because it's such a useful analogy for parenting. Think about it: the two-year-old acts impulsively. She needs to be reminded the stove is hot, to stay out of the street, to keep peas out of her nose. The toddler says "no" as a matter of habit. He challenges limits, wants to "do it myself" and requires frequent naps to keep from spinning out of control. I don't know about you, but my husband and I can say the same about our teenagers.

Thinking about our adolescent children as overgrown, smelly versions of their toddler selves has been immeasurably helpful to our family. A brilliant therapist has guided every single one of us—and all of us together—through this wilderness of adolescent rebellion. One of the most valuable tools she gave us was the reminder of how much teenagers are like two-year-olds. When we call to mind this simple equation, my husband I laugh more. When he remembers that toddlers can't be expected to focus on an entire round of golf, Daddy finds humor in the 15-year-old collapsing into giggles on the eleventh tee box. (It is all very confusing, remember, because adolescence is indeed a regression. This same child played golf with the attention span of a PGA veteran when he was seven years old. My husband had to adjust his expectations, which can confound the best of us.)

When we recall how toddlers forget to flush the toilet and brush their teeth and pick up their toys, these teenagers make more sense. Surely you would not entrust a two-year-old with the responsibility of remembering her lunch or the many components of his baseball uniform or to deliver an important message to her teacher. So when my teenager loses yet another phone or fails to turn in yet another project I know he completed, it is helpful and amusing to remember the toddler brain at work. We don't give up on the idea of a two-year-old eventually maturing. We know she will someday become more responsible and independent. We keep pinning notes to backs and delivering forgotten lunches, knowing it's just a phase. It's the same deal with teenagers, only they're way less cute and their meltdowns are kind of scary.

Even the teenagers themselves—in my own family and in the class-room—are served by the analogy. They cannot escape the accuracy: they really are a lot like toddlers. This knowledge can be a great asset to communication. We have—to great effect—taken a child by the hand and said, "Hey, Little Buddy, let me show you again how we throw our clothes into the hamper and not on the floor. I know you can't remember because you're really only two, so let's just have another lesson." This approach inevitably cracks up the teenager in question. It has also netted more consistent results than my instinctive response, which is to whirl about like a Tasmanian devil, leaving everyone in my path frightened and exhausted. A a sense of humor and shared laughter with our children are healthy antidotes to the teenaged attitude. Acknowledging their toddler tendencies has been a great help in the process.

THEY'RE LESS ADORABLE AND WAY, WAY SCARIER.

Yes, teenagers are like overgrown toddlers, and we do best to raise them with as much love and vigilance as we do our two-year-olds. If a toddler were in the middle of a busy street, any one of us would risk life and limb to save him. If that same child, however, 13 years later, is in the middle of a busy street—especially if his jeans are hanging below his underpants and the bass from his headphones shakes our bones—many of us might swerve out of our way to run him over on purpose. When a toddler enters a shop she endears the proprietor, who gives her a free cookie, a friendly smile, a toy to entertain her when she gets fussy. When that same sweet thing walks into the same shop at 15 years old dressed (on purpose) like a freak of nature, the shopkeeper is likely to activate security cameras and stash baskets of small items under the counter. Society assumes the worst about teenagers. We think they are up to no good. And, honestly, they often are.

Parents (and other adults) delight in watching a toddler explore her world and test her limits. When she stumbles and falls, we murmur soothingly, pick her up, dust her off, and set her on her way again. Because it's all so adorable. Teenagers do the same thing. They test their own limits and our boundaries. They are figuring out who they are in relation to all the other people and things out there in the world. And the world tends to answer with a litany of parental nightmares. When a toddler stumbles, she may skin her knee. When a teenager stumbles, the consequences can be far more serious.

Parents and teachers (and villagers raising our children together) serve our teenagers best when we agree to love them as if they were toddlers. We can give them freedom within boundaries so they can test their own limits. We can step in—sometimes risking life and limb—to rip them away from imminent danger. When they stumble and fall, we can murmur soothingly, pick them up, dust them off, and send them on their way again. Even when it is not even remotely adorable.

Since my children have turned on me and made life crazy, I have endeavored to spend as much time with actual toddlers as possible. I recommend it for all parents of adolescents. First of all, toddlers do smell better—and they are cuter, and easier to distract when they throw tantrums—than teenagers. Secondly, they remind you of a time when you—like Mama Bear—had a better idea of what to do for your kids. When a three-year-old skins her knee, she needs a kiss and an encouraging word. When he melts down in the middle of the sidewalk, he needs a nap. No matter how clever they are, toddlers can't convince us they should eat ice cream for every meal. Hanging out with them is also healthy because their rebellion seems more reasonable than it will 10 years into the future. And as we watch toddlers explore the world and test their limits, we might gain some understanding of our teenagers.

PARENTING CASE STUDY:
The Tale of the Playground Slide

Just the other day, for example, I took one of my favorite little girls to the park. On the longish walk to the playground, she asked me to walk behind her instead of holding her hand. As she approached the tallest slide, she soberly handed me her stuffed dog and began to climb. She shunned my attempts to help her—I can do it myself!—and carefully negotiated her way up the ladder. I nervously spotted her as well as I could without her knowing and soon she was quite out of my reach. As she climbed high above my head I was struck by how apt a metaphor the moment was for the whole parenting enchilada. If she tumbled from her happy perch so high above me, I would be hard-pressed to help her. I knew it and perhaps she knew it, too. If I had stopped her from climbing too high, however, it would have been like clipping her wings, thwarting her independence. Again, that half-second parenting conundrum!

Instead of fretting or telegraphing my un-ease, I tried to shout encouraging things to my toddler friend. I asked if she was proud of herself. She was! Very! I asked if she wanted to come down soon. She did not! I offered to join her if she wanted company. No, thank you! She sat at the tippy-top of the playground climber, gazing out at the world, narrating her own little reverie, calling down to me occasionally just to be sure I was still paying attention. At one point she sang the entire Lollipop Guild song from *The Wizard of Oz* at the top of her lungs. Eventually, she came barreling down the corkscrew slide, laughing and breathless from her adventure. As we left, she paused to look back at the mountain of her accomplishment. "I climbed to the top. All by myself!

Mommy will be so excited!" And she let me hold her hand part of the way home.

. . . .

That moment at the playground—suspended in time and conflicted emotions—when toddlers climb out of our grasp is a premonition of the teenaged years. As they clamber beyond our reach we are scared but we know we have to let them do it. The sense of accomplishment they earn is worth the risk. Why is climbing to the top of the slide so important? Why is anything worth the risk of bodily harm? Because it is their job to develop coping skills. To learn resilience and self-regulation. And it's our job as parents to facilitate the whole amazing (frustrating, scary, mind-numbing) process. I promise, when they grow up to be people we actually like, who do well and do good in the world, Mommy will be so excited, indeed!

Parents can seize the opportunity of the plastic, malleable, open-window teenaged brain. We can keep our teenagers relatively safe from harm if we know them, protect them and honor them. It may take everything we've got, but our kids and our families are worth it. If we can parent with open eyes, strong arms and full hearts, maybe we can all survive these crazy years intact.

MEET THEM WHERE THEY ARE.

As important as it is to protect our teenagers, it is at least as vital to honor their development, their process and their foibles. They learn to regulate by being regulated, which looks different than parents making every decision for them. We seek to gradually decrease our support as they grow up. When our children are adolescents, it is difficult to find the balance. There's a fine line between helping them and doing things for them. There's a fine line between challenging them and abandoning them. Teachers have long sought to work within a child's *zone of proximal development*: the space between what students can do independently and what they can do with assistance. (Vygotsky, 1934) It's the ideal place for learning to happen. To successfully work within a student's zone of proximal development, teachers need to know where children are functioning today, where they may be functioning tomorrow, and how to help them master more advanced skills and concepts. The zone of proximal development, however, is not a comfortable space to be.

Students (and three-year-olds) learning new skills are often frustrated. If they learn to work through their discomfort, they can meet new demands and challenges with a sense of confidence. This seems important to me as a parent, because meeting new demands and challenges is a pretty big part of adult life. When they learn to rely on themselves—when they know they can do hard things, survive, and even triumph—there's no stopping them in adulthood. But—once again—it's a fine, fine line.

You know the feeling of being completely frustrated by something you thought you couldn't do? I remember standing at the top of a mountain when I was about 11 years old, crying and screaming at my father because I didn't think I could ski down it. I was scared. I was panicked. Eventually I figured out a way to stop crying and get down. It wasn't pretty, but I wasn't dead, either, and that particular mogul run lost its mythic power. It never frightened me quite as much again. There's that zone of proximal development. Kids learn in stages and we help. Often, we help them work through frustration and breathe through fear. It can be unpleasant, watching our kids struggle and feel uncomfortable. But if tasks don't get more demanding, there will be no learning, no growth. The tasks of adolescence are very demanding.

Here's another benefit of those malleable, developing, adolescent brains: meeting challenges in the present helps the brain establish connections which will help meet challenges in the future (Steinberg, 2014). The act of working and breathing through frustration now helps prepare the brain to handle setbacks in adult life. Working within the zone of proximal development is more beneficial than performing the same easy tasks over and over again. The new adolescent brain science promises that scaffolding—challenging our kids within their zone of proximal development—actually builds stronger prefrontal systems in their brains. I just love it when science and common-sense come together.

Yes, adolescents are slaves to the chemical experiments Mother Nature is conducting in their bodies. Their wiring makes it tough to control impulses or resist peer pressure or care much at all about long-term consequences. Teenagers are the new toddlers. The good news is, this time in their development is a great opportunity for parents to make a positive difference in who they will become.

The other good news is this: it gets better. *It gets better.* The toddlers do grow up. The teenager's brains mature. In most cases, they act human again eventually (even to us). In the meantime, we need to stay alert and pay attention, because the road toward adulthood leads our teenagers through dangerous territory. So much threatens to knock them right off the path toward becoming healthy, happy, responsible adults. As crazy as they make their parents during this decade or so, it is vital we try to keep them safe and not give up on them now.

Chapter Six

Go Back to the Beginning: What Do We Really Want for Our Children?

May you teach them about enough of society's conventions that
they can survive, but not so much that they are imprisoned.
~Dan Pashmin, *The Sporkful* Podcast

PARENTS CAN'T RELY on a clear description of our jobs; there are no operating instructions for human children. Relying on others' definitions of parenting leads us down the primrose path. The job changes perpetually anyway (as per the natural functions of adolescence and family life). If we can't exactly define what we're doing, how the heck do we plan our days? With all the teenaged drama marring our vision, how on God's green earth can we see the forest for the trees? Here is where my years in education come in handy. We must begin with the end in mind. Teachers plan their curriculum, lessons and day-to-day operations according to what they want students to know and do by the end of the year. As promised, I will show you new ways of looking at teenagers and how to raise them. Here is one important shift in perspective: let's also look at our children from a distant, future point of view. As we begin to contemplate solutions to what seems like an unresolvable problem, (adolescence!) we do best to think about the outcomes we desire.

Teachers discuss backward planning and outcomes for instruction (Wiggins & McTighe, 2005) and all of us know instinctively what these terms mean. We plan backward when we cook a meal, get to a destination or build a bookshelf. To one degree or another, we begin with the outcome. We think, "I'd like lasagna for dinner" or "I need to visit my mother" or "a bookshelf would be great in this corner." We make a plan and accomplish the task according to the result we have in mind. We boil noodles if we want lasagna; we don't throw a chicken into the oven. One cook might follow an old family recipe from memory; another may consult a celebrity chef's website for inspiration; still others will improvise according to what's in the fridge. Ingredients and techniques may vary, but if we want that lasagna, we begin with noodles and tomato sauce. As we grate mozzarella and sauté onions, we take steps to manifest the outcome we desire: a pan of lasagna on the table at dinnertime. On the drive to Mom's house, we may wander, take a circuitous route or run errands along the way, but we know our final destination and we head in that general direction. Likewise, the final shape we envision for our bookshelf will determine the materials we need to get started. Probably we will measure the corner, cut wood to specific lengths and buy an assortment of screws and nails. We plan backward every day, all day long. It's almost inconceivable not to do so: how would we begin to build a shelf we had not yet imagined? When it comes to parenting, it's a similar thing. We likely began with some ideas—no matter how vague or expansive—of what we wanted for our children, but by the time they hit puberty, we are often too exhausted to remember. The muck and mire of daily existence clouds the visions, hopes and dreams we once had for our children.

I have asked you to try and remember your teenagers as they were when they were toddlers. Now let's go back even further. Take a moment and recall the sweet brand-new smell of your infant son or daughter. When we carried little car seats across the threshold to establish our families, the future looked bright indeed. The illimitable promise of a tiny baby is overwhelming (especially when that baby is yours). Oh, sure, it's terrifying: the responsibility, the expense, the absurdity of this new person entrusted entirely to us! But who among us can count the joyful hours we lost cooing and whispering into a little newborn face? I distinctly remember rocking my first born during his second month, meditating on the graceful curve of his ear while his father sat nearby in similar adoration. In the dim nursery light we gazed into the future: maybe he will love golf or football! Maybe he'll be an investment banker or a farmer or a priest. Maybe he'll become a philanthropist and change the course of human history! Or maybe he'll just like to knit sweaters. Every single thing we can fathom for a baby seems quite literally possible and—as long as the reverie doesn't include anything too negative—we're okay with all of it. (I remember too in that moment knowing every other parent in the history of time had felt the same way: the mothers and fathers of saints and martyrs, kings and murderers. It was humbling, the mundanity of our personal miracle.)

When our parenting hearts are this full our dreams are simple and spacious. We want our children to be happy. We hope they will enjoy their time on the big blue marble. We hope they will feel loved and useful and full of joy. We hope they will do well in the world and we hope they will do good. We can't really imagine what shape they will take nor which course they will chart and we don't much care. We know with everything we have how amazing, beautiful and possibly enchanted our children are; we trust the universe will respond appropriately. We worry less at this stage about ACT scores or which medical school they attend. We care less about which scumbag friends they bring home or what hideous video game they want to play. Backward planning for little children—what we wish for their futures—is painted with broad, happy strokes.

65

Somewhere along the line (I blame the puberty hormones), we lose this sunny perspective and forget our goals.

So let's think about this: what do we really want for our children? Not the details so menacing during adolescence—specific coursework or hobbies, curfews or clubs, colleges or career choices—the big stuff. Assuming the world will look a little different when they are adults, what do we really want for them? What do we want them to be? To have? To do? As we consider the enormity of these questions, Rousseau (the godfather of modern education) comes to mind again. An enthusiastic champion of inherent human goodness, Rousseau believes it is our job to help keep each (perfect) child intact despite the injuries of the cruel world. Society threatens at every turn to corrupt innocence and purity, Rousseau insists; rearing children means helping them survive unscathed. He describes the task of teaching them how to stay true to their fundamental integrity as they face all those slings, arrows, outrageous fortunes and what-have-you (1762). Assuming we don't intend to cloister our progeny, how do we do that? How can we keep them whole while we expose them to the broken world?

Well, we can give them tools of resistance. We can equip them to stay strong against temptation, torment and treachery. In the world of constant media messaging, these survival tools are more vital than ever. The shape those tools take—like lesson plans and scaffolding techniques in the class-room—matters less than the outcomes we want. How we reach our goals and measure those outcomes will be different for each child and each parent, but the outcomes themselves are pretty universal.

Yes, they should be able to launder clothes and make a few meals, change a tire and pay taxes. Maybe I want my kids to know how to write a thank-you note, tell a joke or play piano. We may feel like failures if they can't survive on their own in the wilderness, do a back-flip, make clever small talk at parties or list the entire Beatles catalog from memory. We want a lot of things for our kids but it's all small stuff. Life entails more details than we can address. So many unexpected things will be demanded of our children once they become adults, we can't prepare them for the specifics. We've got to look at the big picture, the essential understandings they need to navigate the world. In terms of skills and outcomes, what should our kids be able to do at the end of their time in our care? Adolescents will soon be making decisions about where they spend their money, whom they support in elections, and how they conduct themselves in the wide, weird world. Although our job is difficult to define, we can discuss the results we want. So many not-important things get in the way it's hard to focus on the real tasks of the family system during adolescence, but let's give it a shot.

Here's my list. These are five things I hope my children will be able to do when they are no longer in my care. These are qualities I admire in other adults and wish I had more of myself. See how my list compares to yours.

. . . .

Five Things I Hope My Children Will Be Able to Do When They Leave My House:

1. See the Good in the World

Life is hard but worth it. I say this so much to teenagers they roll their eyes when they hear it. I repeat it, to them and to myself, because it's so true and so important. It's easy to succumb to the struggle, especially for teenagers; immediacy is their jam. It's easy to get mired in the ugliness of existence. I hope my children will grow up to be people who rise above it. Who see the pain but focus on the joy. No matter how we wish we could sequester them from reality, our kids will see some pretty rough stuff. Call it what you will—a glass-half-full personality, a sunny disposition, a Pollyanna persona—I want my kids to have a positive view of the world. I want them to see the world with open eyes. All of it, flaws and foibles. And I want them to see the silver lining in every cloud. [2]

2. Manifest Change for Themselves and Others

People who can see good in the world also tend to trust their ability to affect change when it is needed. How often adults—all of us—curse the darkness instead of lighting a candle! I want my children to have what sociologists call an *interior locus of control*: the perception of responsibility for their own life and actions. People who believe outside forces are responsible for all their misfortunes and successes tend to feel victimized by circumstance. Those who believe the course of their lives is at least partly a result of their own doing, on the other hand, can manifest change. They can get themselves out of ruts, awful situations and complex challenges. First, they have a view of the world positive enough to envision change. Then, they call upon their inner strength to make the change. They think outside the box. They seek solutions instead of whining about problems. They survive and thrive. They're nice people to be around. I hope my children become adults who don't feel like victims. I hope they find ways to help themselves—and others—feast on life's banquet.

3. Maintain a Healthy Body

One undeniable task of adolescence is to physically mature. To grow up. Part of our job is keeping kids safe and healthy enough to reach the pinnacle of adulthood. With this outcome in mind parents can see clearly the importance of rest, exercise, good nutrition and keeping kids away from drugs and alcohol. At the end of the road—when they are fully grown themselves—I hope my kids will know how to make choices to stay healthy.

As we have observed, the adolescent brain is malleable, plastic, an open window, predisposed to seek and sense pleasure. Teenagers are responsive to outside stimuli and their brains form according to how they experience the world. Regular pleasure from drugs and alcohol—and conversely, regular pleasure from exercise and engaging hobbies—wires the brain for future experience. It is the parents' job to provide a healthy environment for this development, while scaffolding the process so they know how to create and maintain healthy adult environments for themselves.

4. Establish a Unique Identity

I am not you; you are not me. These are words we should repeat to ourselves like a mantra during the painful process of adolescent identity formation. Since the dawn of time wisdom tells us it is each child's task to establish autonomy from the family of origin. As I've gone on and on about already, the act itself is violent and painful. But it's one of the most important parts of growing up into responsible adulthood. Our kids have to figure out who they are apart from us.

We nudge kids in the direction of independence by gradually helping them become more responsible for their own decision-making. They need to feel secure in our support and guidance while they reject and condemn our very presence in their lives. Their identity crisis is a good thing, remember. It eventually allows them to make commitments, choose careers and remain true to themselves when the storms of existence blow like a hurricane. When all is said and done (and they're no longer living in our home) I hope my children will know who they are. I hope they will have an unshakable sense of self, anchored in our family but open to experience. With a positive world view, a strong interior locus of control, a healthy brain and a solid sense of identity, kids grow up to do just as I labored to teach my students. They think for themselves. They know who they are. They read and watch with healthy skepticism. They have an internal shelter from the storms of life.

5. Self-Regulate

I want my kids to be able to commit to and complete a task. I want them to believe hard work pays off. I want them to be capable of focusing on the future instead of only on the present. Life's banquet dishes up plenty of opportunities to delay gratification, to do things we'd rather not do in order to reap later benefits. Self-regulation is the ability to envision those future rewards, wait for them and work for them. The brain circuits regulating self-control are strengthened during adolescence. We need to help our kids with these skills now (because they are hormonal messes) and gradually let them practice on their own. By scaffolding their journey toward independence, we can help self-regulation be more automatic—and much easier—for them when they are adults. It's a lifelong struggle to delay gratification and make responsible choices, but the way we learn to do it in adolescence can make a big difference in how easily it comes later in life.

Tenacity almost always trumps raw talent. If my children can rely on the executive functions of their brains (decision-making, problem-solving, planning ahead) as well as their natural gifts, there will be no end to the richness of their lives.

During the adolescent years it's best not to worry so much about what jobs they'll work or whom they will marry. We can instead envision qualities we admire in adults: a positive attitude, intrepid spirit and good health. We can think of people we know who seem self-confident but not cocky, who find a balance between work and play, who are curious and intelligent. When we name the things we want our children to be able to do, the amorphous job of parenting starts to take shape. Articulating these outcomes is important because it helps us keep our eye on the prize, even amidst the noise and commotion of the three-ring circus we call family life. Goals, statements of tasks and measurable objectives also allow us to check in along the way. Even daily—when teenagers are making mischief of one kind or another—we can see how we're doing. Keeping the big objectives in mind helps us turn down the volume on less important things. The outcomes we want for our children help us remember why the daily grind is worth it in the end.

As we delve further into how to accomplish this lofty goal (completing the tasks of adolescence) let's remember how vital it is to stay vigilant. Our work is too important now to fall asleep on the job. Our adolescent children need us in new, confusing, challenging ways. Parents with open eyes know what's going on with their kids. Parents with strong arms can protect their teens from any real and present danger. Parents with full hearts can honor each personal, different-from-ours journey toward adulthood. I repeat: it is exhausting. Staying on top of our kids while maneuvering around their mercurial moods and reactions is an ugly, painful, messy process. If we keep the end in mind, it all makes a little more sense.

. . . .

PARENTING CASE STUDY:
God Bless the Child That's Got His Own.

One summer our 15-year-old son disappeared into the airport security crowd. I watched him walk—backpack over his shoulder, confident but frightened, excited but anxious—in the direction of his dreams. He was heading for a summer of commercial salmon fishing in Alaska, a place none of us had ever been. We knew we wouldn't see him for six weeks. (We didn't know how rarely we would hear from him.) We knew he longed for this adventure and we knew it was best to let him go. But I am his mother and as he walked out of my sight at the airport, I cried.

I would miss him and I was apprehensive, but as he slipped into the sea of airport humanity my tears fell for another reason altogether: I knew he was going to be okay. I knew in my gut as he left that he's got what it takes. He is strong and resilient and smart. He's gutsy and intrepid and most of the time he makes really, really good choices. I am still amazed by his willingness to face (to fly right into!) the unknown. I am overcome equally with pride and humility; despite our parental mistakes and weaknesses, our child has got his own.

For me, those six weeks were a season of waiting, of trusting, of not knowing, of missing my boy. A season of thinking good thoughts and hoping for no news (because it always means good news). And then our child came home. Bearded and filthy and happy. Different. Grown-up. Many times we've seen evidence of the perspective he gained, being lonely and working hard and living among strangers. He is a man of few words and we saw only a few photographs of his entire experience, which means most of it belongs only to him.

It is a beautiful mystery watching our children do things completely unknown to us. Only when we let them go (sometimes miles and time zones away, into the literal wilderness) do we give them the space and the freedom to become themselves.

Chapter Seven

Rock and a Hard Place: Why Parenting Teenagers Feels So Impossible

So I'm supposed to pump him up
but not so much that he's afraid to let me down?
It's ironic that I'm struggling with this since my greatest
cheerleading move was Threading the Needle.
~Phil Dunphy, *Modern Family*

· ·

PARENTING CASE STUDY:
A Teenager's Two-Fold Lament

Melody spent the entire lunch period sobbing in my classroom. Finals and graduation loomed but Mel was generally excited about her future; she had signed to play lacrosse and study at a top-notch university (achievements, by the by, which do not generally come without years of parental support and sacrifice). She was a disciplined, popular, happy-go-lucky girl; until she broke down at my desk, I had never seen her so much as scowl.

"My parents are so humiliating," she cried. "All they ever do is brag about me. I can't stand it!" A litany of parental affronts tumbled out with her tears: they cheer too loudly at games; they take credit for her accomplishments; they have her jersey number on a bumper sticker! Mom posts pictures on Facebook of every out-of-town game and she hung a booster club flag from the front porch on signing day! They just make such a big deal about everything. Even grandparents, when they call, want to hear all about Melody's season, her teammates and her stats. "It's so annoying," Mel repeated over and over. "My dad actually cut an article about me out of the newspaper and sent it to his dumb old fraternity friend." She continued: "I'm honestly not even that good at lacrosse. I mean, lots of people are better than me! They act like I'm so special and it's all they ever talk about."

As Melody cursed her parents' inflated view of her accomplishments, her rant took an unexpected turn. "And also? I can never ever do anything right," she wept. "Nothing I do is ever good enough." Out poured a new list of indignities: "All they ever do is tell me how lame I am. They think I'm stupid and they don't trust me and they don't even act like they care." Offenses in this category included not making a big enough deal about Melody's upcoming graduation party and failing to show up with an armful of roses at the Prom fashion show. "Every other dad came onstage at the end and handed his daughter a huge bouquet," Melody explained. "Except mine. All I got was a hug. It was so humiliating." She continued, "I work really hard and I'm really successful but all my parents see is when I screw up. They only notice when I lose something or miss curfew and it's all they ever talk about."

Parents, we cannot win. Melody's complaints illuminate our position: we are stuck precisely between a rock and a hard place. If we hold them too closely our children bristle but they resent it when we give them too much space. We all know the phrase "cutting the apron strings" and (intellectually) we get it. Kids need to break away. They need to test their independence, differentiate from us, get used to living without our care. It is an inherently painful process. But "cutting the apron strings" is far too gentle a metaphor to explain the process. The image conjures Donna Reed and *Father Knows Best* and even *The Brady Bunch*—apron-wearing, advice-dispensing parents finding tidy solutions for their teen-agers' quirky problems, all within a jovial half-hour. I don't know about you, but that's not how it generally feels at our house.

One of our parental tasks is to help children structure, define and nego-tiate the universe. It's easier when they are younger because we enjoy our roles and because their interests are pretty adorable. As little ones develop unique personalities before our very eyes, we want to nurture their individual passions and predilections. When a preschooler develops an obsession with Disney princesses or the Ninja Turtles, it's easier to indulge than when the same kid—a decade later—spends every Friday night at Hot Topic or plugged into death metal. My husband and I supple-mented our kindergartener's all-consuming passion for bats (the flying rodent variety) with every book we could find, weekly trips to the zoo and handcrafted Halloween costumes. When our three-year-old friends imagine they are surrounded by lions (or whales or monkeys), adults don't think twice about crawling around on all fours making animal noises as they order us to sit, roll over and chase them. Many families we know have made vacation-pilgrimages to places like the Baseball Hall of Fame or American Girl Place! Every new discovery our kids make, every new friend they meet, every new skill amazes and delights us. It is less joyful (and more frightening) when our teens start quoting full episodes of *Trailer Park Boys* and mounting arguments on their desire for a tribal tattoo. Aggressively loud, rabidly hungry strangers who barely look you in the eye will send you running for cover in your own home.

It's not just that their hobbies and personalities change. It's how often (and violently and unpredictably) they change. My 13-year-old niece was an ardent fan of what I call the hipster bacon movement (when stores were stocked with a ready supply of bacon bandages, bacon-flavored soda and tuxedos made of plastic bacon). She flooded her Instagram account with bacon-themed memes and postures. "Life is better with bacon" was her motto during the summer months as she experimented with recipes for every occasion. By Christmastime—with no fanfare at all—the child was a vegan. Her devoted family didn't get the memo and lovingly filled her stocking with cured meat in every form. When she turned up her nose in disgust, they didn't get it. When she pouted about the existential indignity of being misunderstood by *everybody*, her loved ones were flummoxed and somehow disappointed in themselves.

And so. Inspired by the habits of parents I admire, who find a delicate balance on the high wire of raising teenagers, who know, protect and honor their offspring, I give you our new role models. We live in hope!

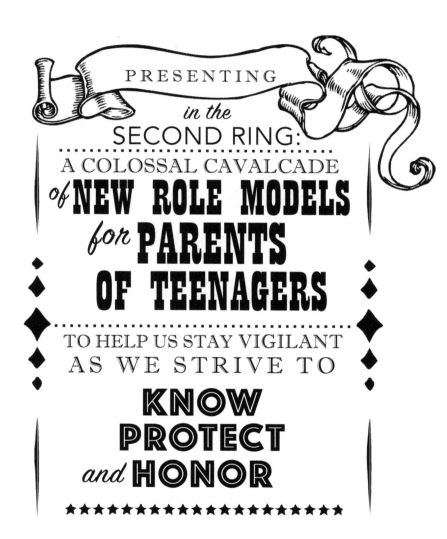

PRESENTING

in the
SECOND RING:
A COLOSSAL CAVALCADE
of NEW ROLE MODELS
for PARENTS
OF TEENAGERS

TO HELP US STAY VIGILANT
AS WE STRIVE TO

KNOW
PROTECT
and HONOR

ROLE MODELS
WHO KNOW

THE PEREGRINE FALCON
THE PRIVATE INVESTIGATOR
THE NINJA

Chapter Eight

Peregrine Falcon
(Watch Them)

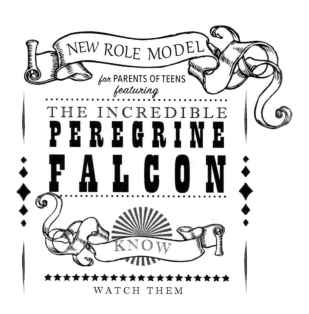

SHORTLY AFTER I decided Mama Bear (and all her hibernating) would no longer serve as my parenting role model, I caught a Discovery Channel show about the peregrine falcon. The mother falcon leaves her chicks in the nest when she flies off to hunt. She lets them fend for themselves as far as their young age allows. She seems not to worry about choking hazards (or SAT scores), but when the danger gets real, this Mama doesn't play. When giant pelicans fly too near her cliffside nest, Mother Falcon swoops in (at over 200 miles per hour!) to save those babies. She knocks her enemies right out of the sky. The pelicans drop awkwardly into the ocean. She checks the nest, sees her chicks are safe, and flies back again to her business. As I watched the drama unfold, I thought, *"This* is the kind of parent I want to be!"

Ladies and Gentlemen, my original new role model for parents of teens: Mother Peregrine Falcon. I long to know my parenting priorities as well as she. I too want to trust my children's ability to survive the injurious world with their own strengths and skills. But when very real predators threaten my teenagers, may I have the good sense to swoop in and save them.

BIRD'S-EYE VIEW: KNOW THE REALITY OF TEENAGERS.

Mother Falcon keeps a healthy distance from her young brood. No "helicoptering" or "Tiger-Mom" for her; she's got a life of her own and she tends to it. But always, always, always, this mother bird has a steely eye trained on her chicks. She knows they're rather helpless but she also knows it's their job to become independent. So she flies off and lets them struggle a little bit. She doesn't freak out when her fledglings crane their necks precariously toward the world beyond the nest. Talk about a mom who's got her priorities in order! She doesn't sweat the small stuff. She sees it all and takes action only when absolutely necessary.

So how do we know when it's absolutely necessary? How do we discern the difference between normal teenaged drama and life-threatening danger? How can we parent like Mother Falcon, who seems instinctively to know the difference?

Well, my friends, here we are again at the heart of the matter. It's a very fine line. It's a three-ring circus of unexpected situations and parents need to be nimble and creative in our responses. We need to be prepared for the unexpected, ready to pivot at any time. Every child, every challenge requires us to step back and assess the situation. Only when we know our children well can we make educated, sound, helpful choices in our parenting. Our new role models, starting with the Falcon, can guide us. We can also turn to teachers and other adults to help us get to know our kids.

Three Ways Teachers Can Help You KNOW Who Your Teenagers Really Are

1. Let Teenagers Make Their Own First Impressions.
Well-meaning parents sell their teenagers short by sticking labels on them. Teachers know the power of the Pygmalion Effect and its ugly cousin the Golem Effect, the blessing/curse of self-fulfilling prophesy in the classroom. Generations of research has shown teachers perform differently with students for whom they have high expectations. They are better teachers—and the classroom climate is more productive—for these students than those for whom they have low expectations. Parents who label can unwittingly set a low bar and negatively influence a teacher's first impressions of their child.

Often teachers receive emails—from parents, tutors, mentors or other specialists—detailing the learning challenges their student faces and the modifications needed for her to prosper in school. Some of these emails, of course, contain physical, emotional and processing requirements which teachers must follow to the letter (and to the law). Many times, though, the information creates a slight and unnecessary Golem Effect between the teacher and the kid in question.

Parents seeking to protect their children from the overwhelming world of high school (or varsity baseball, or any new and scary situation) drop helpful hints to adults about their child's social or physical awkwardness, difficulties paying attention, or test-taking challenges. Time and again, these comments do not resemble the child who shows up to class. I think parents do better when they let teachers discover who their children are; even better, parents who listen to a teacher's perspective can gain valuable insights.

2. Listen to What Others Say about Your Teenager.
Reportedly shy teenagers might hold animated conversations in the classroom. The student with chronic dyslexia might prove herself a savant—and the envy of her peers—when it comes to diagramming sentences. The perennial behavior problem may perform beautifully for a teacher who recognizes his innate ability to translate diction into tone. On the other hand, the former book-worm may delight in devising creative ways to cause pandemonium in class. Your darling angel may, indeed, be leaving campus at lunch to smoke weed in the park. The truth hurts, but we fail our children when we don't listen to it and act accordingly.

Believe it or not, teachers want every student to win, to get it, to score well on the final, to care deeply about learning. When teachers meet a new class, we are excited to discover the possibilities and potential of our new students. Every time we grade a stack of tests, we root for each kid to hit it out of the park. We feel like superheroes when they do well; we sadly blame ourselves when it goes otherwise. Parents with the best intentions can damage a teacher's goodwill toward a student with outdated, inaccurate, or limiting labels.

3. Suck it up and Go to Parent-Teacher Conferences.

Standing in lines all afternoon may seem obsolete in this age of 24-hour access to the gradebook, but conferences are a great resource for parents who want to know their teenagers. Go. I urge you. Go; open your ears and your heart. I assure you, teachers can give us valuable information about our children. Try to bite your tongue and tell teachers less about your kids. Try to listen instead, to stories about who your children really are—how they act, what they say, who influences them—and let this new knowledge help you see your adolescents with new eyes.

. . . .

Chapter Nine

Private Investigator
(Study Them)

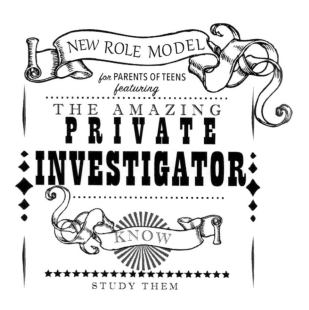

THE PARENTS I have studied (because I want to emulate their methods) don't hibernate. They stay vigilant and study their teenagers. They know their kids. They pay attention. If we hope to maintain our balance on the high wire of parenting adolescents, we need to really know what's going on. Only then can we determine when to pick our teenagers up (because they are in real danger) and when to let them fall (because they will learn best from real consequences).

Like hired detectives, these parents keep track of clues in order to solve a mystery. Teenagers themselves leave the clues, both consciously and haphazardly. Knowing our teenagers means studying them. Gathering intel. Figuring out what makes them tick, who influences them and what they're up to when they think we're not looking. Our next new role model for parenting teenagers, then, is the Private Investigator.

SHOULD I TRUST MY TEENAGER?

At a certain point in Mother Nature's little *commedia*, the fruits of our loins cannot be trusted. Some teenagers lie for sport; others are simply incapable of expressing the truth thanks to hormones (they can't make sense of any danged thing). It's up to you how much trust you extend. Many parents belong to the "trust, but verify" school, which I think mostly makes sense. It's probably ideal to trust everyone but brand our own cattle, so to speak. But personally—and until further notice—I don't trust teenagers any further than I can throw 'em. (It's not personal. It's not permanent. And it's not their fault. Remember: I am quite familiar with the teenaged brain.)

As always, we walk a fine line. Of course it makes sense much of the time to trust our kids and let them make their own choices. Often it is imperative to let them fail and face their consequences. Most of the time they do just fine. But (oh, that teenaged brain!) they are predisposed to acting recklessly and taking risks. Their grasp of cause and effect is tenuous; they're being poisoned by hormones. We try to strike a balance as magical and ephemeral as spun sugar: to give teenagers freedom to be themselves (their messy, imperfect, full-of-contradiction selves) while maintaining boundaries to keep them safe.

Doing investigative work feels wrong to many parents because it seems so invasive. We worry they won't trust us if we appear not to trust them. I must admit, I'm not terribly concerned about how much kids trust me during their adolescent years. I have learned not to listen when they describe me; that way lies madness. Still, it's a fine line between knowing what's going on with them and invading their privacy.

Gradually, developmentally, teenagers force the privacy issue. They close doors and stop talking and plug into headphones (even in polite company). Family patterns naturally evolve in response and we know much less about their daily lives than we once did. All this behavior is appropriate, even necessary. But privacy can turn quickly into secrecy, which can put teenagers in real danger. In a perfect world, we'd leave them to themselves to develop and mature. But in this imperfect world, a little less privacy may save our children.

While walking this tightrope, the parents I admire err on the side of knowledge. They don't hover but they learn what's going on. Behind the scenes, surreptitiously, like private investigators, they clean messy bedrooms, go through pockets, read journals, run hands between mattresses, strip beds, borrow cars (for the express purpose of sifting through glove compartments), check bank accounts and monitor technology. They know the influences so strong in their children's lives; they gather solid intelligence.

Parents who study their kids in this fashion reap two benefits. First of all, they know enough to discern when a kid is in real trouble. They can suss out the difference between normal teenaged drama and actual, imminent danger. Second, they have the deep and abiding pleasure of being surprised by the good their kids are up to. They collect clues about behavior and make notes. Often, when the big picture comes into focus, we see an awful lot of beauty in our teens. (Don't get me wrong: we also see heaps and heaps of dumbass. But not every discovery the private investigator makes deserves a response. For now, we're just quietly gathering data.)

. . . .

Nine Things You Might Have to Do to Study Your Teens like a P.I.

1. Crawl through bushes

...or drive out of your way or place a call to someone you barely know at an inappropriate hour. Just to make sure everybody is where they're supposed to be.

2. Feel uncomfortable

...because teenagers can get the upper hand—and develop secret, dangerous habits—when parents feel uncomfortable. Some of us feel awkward or invasive introducing ourselves to parents of our kids' friends. I'm begging you to suck it up, bake some banana bread if that helps you, and make the introduction. Show up on the doorstep of your daughter's boyfriend's home. Say, "Our kids are spending a lot of time together and I thought we should know each other a little bit." What parents who love and care about their own children could possibly take offense? Your teenagers don't need to know about any of these actions, by the way, and certainly we don't need their permission. A private investigator operates under the radar whenever possible.

3. Suffer through a concert

...because you trust your kid but you don't trust the crowd. So you say yes, he can go, but you will also be there. You will wear earplugs and you will stand at the back, but you will be there. Watching. Studying.

4. Conduct research

...to understand them. When the kids are talking about sizzurp or mollys, urbandictionary.com is your first among many online resources. When kids sound like they're talking in code, crack it. We have the whole worldwide web at our fingertips: get online and decipher the meaning of their adolescent ramblings.

Doing our research also lets us see when our teenagers are doing good stuff. When a TOK bumper sticker on the car of your friend's daughter alerts your radar (TOK? As in toke? Is that a pot reference?) a little internet research might put you at ease. That sticker, in fact, is a badge of honor from the International Baccalaureate Theory of Knowledge course, and a right fine thing for a teenager to display on her ride. Good to know. (I'm not saying I did that research myself. I'm not saying I didn't.)

5. Learn how to use GPS tracking devices

...and all other creative means vigilant parents take to keep track of their kids. Instagram posts at 2:00 AM, secret (and questionable) Pinterest boards, euphemistic tweets, fantasy gaming personae, oh dear heavens, the list is endless indeed. Studying their patterns—both in real life and on social media—keeps us apprised of what teens are doing and where they are.

6. Ask ridiculous questions

...such as: Why are you carrying a lighter in your pocket? What could you possibly have been doing there at three in the morning? What happened to the [fill in the blank with any number of frightening substances missing from household cabinets, freezers and garages]?

Why are you wearing long sleeves and a turtleneck in July? Who is this person? Why are they calling you that? What does this mean?

They don't like it when we ask these questions. Not one little bit. And, indeed, sometimes judicious silence is best. But a heck of a lot of the time, studying our teenagers like a private investigator means continuing to ask questions just like these.

7. Watch really, really stupid movies

...which is harder for some parents than others, but it is imperative to educate ourselves in pop culture. What they think is funny is awful. You know it; I know it; the grown-ups all know it. Try not to dismiss and condemn. Keep the eye-rolling to a minimum. If we don't tune in a little—if we don't watch and listen along with our kids—we miss out on knowing what is shaping them. (Stay the course. Their sense of taste improves significantly every year. Your calculated exposure to classic rock and *Seinfeld* are not in vain.) In the meantime, if your kids beg to show you another absurd and tasteless video, thank your lucky stars they're talking to you, and watch.

Try to encourage, celebrate and be interested in the things that genuinely interest them. Often these are the very things that annoy you, like terrible music and sophomoric humor and dumb movies and questionable websites. Remember how out of touch your parents seemed? Do not be that way. This does not mean acting or trying to be hip. It does not mean dressing like a teenager. It does not (God, no!) mean being their friend. It does mean doing your research and trying to figure them out. What do your kids think is cool and funny, and why? Which influences are innocent and which are harmful? Again, we have the internet and technology at our fingertips; it is easier for us than it was for our parents to stay tuned in.

Instead of writing off all their entertainment as the ruin of modern civilization, plug in just a little. Rest assured, as they get older, the stuff they think is funny becomes actually funny. It might not be your taste, but open your heart and appreciate the clever. Laughing with your kids is tonic to many family struggles. There is also the possibility—if we plug in and laugh with them—that our teenagers will keep talking to us.

8. See them honestly

...parents do best to see the reality of their gangly, awkward (beautiful) teens, including all their faults and foibles. Knowing our teenagers means seeing their tenderness and their beauty and protecting them from anything that truly threatens to harm them.

9. Face the music.

...ay, there's the rub. All this intelligence leads a good detective to solid conclusions. What we learn about our teens—as we study their behavior, their patterns, their influences—might be hard to handle. Resist Mama Bear's instinct to hibernate; decry the mother ostrich, who buries her head in the sand! Look instead to our new role model, the private investigator. Study your subject well and stay neutral. In a clear moment, from a point of detachment, you'll decide your course of action.

· ·

> Never argue with a fool; onlookers may not be able to tell the difference.
>
> ~**Mark Twain**

. . . .

Three Ways to Respond When Teenagers
Try to Shock You

1. The Slow Blink

This is my absolute favorite tactic. It's the perfect technique for avoiding adolescence garbage because it gives you time to take a breath and it visually removes you from the situation. And because I like you, I'm going to walk you through the steps of the perfect parental slow blink. First, let your face go slack. Cultivate no expression at all; activate none of the muscles in your visage. Next, gently close your eyelids. Really close them so the world goes dark, but don't snap them shut or squeeze them tight. Just lightly lower your eyelids until they are closed. Then (with your eyes shut), roll your eyes. Take a good, indulgent, excessive closed-eye roll. Think briefly to yourself how deeply ridiculous your very own child is at this moment. With your eyes still shut, take one last deep breath. Let it out slowly and audibly. Open your eyes. Look at your child. Think briefly to yourself how deeply wonderful your child is at some moments. If you are physically able, walk away.

2. The Walk Away

When your teen is spouting nonsense, quietly remove yourself from the situation. Don't bite the crazy-bait. Don't leave in anger and don't slam doors. Don't mumble anything under your breath. Just leave. If your child pursues you (in anger, panic or desperation), you may say short, reassuring sentences such as, "I love you" or "Let's calm down and discuss this in a couple of hours," but keep walking. Close the door to your bedroom or the bathroom. Remain calm no matter the protest. Refuse to speak to your teenager until emotions have subsided.

3. The Non-Answer
"Oh." "Huh." "Is that right?" "Sure."

When your adolescent son or daughter drops a bomb into conversation, employ one of these non-answers. Whether it's a pronouncement of sexual identity, a rejection of your religion or plans to follow a band all summer and live in a van, do not react in any logical way. Do not succumb to a teenager's attempts to shock you. Respond first with a non-answer, a profound lack of emotion, and a few follow-up questions if you feel ready. "Tell me more." "Oh, really? What brings you to this conclusion?" If your kid plays along and discusses some goofy idea or plan, play along right back. Do not under any circumstance talk logically ("How do you plan to afford that?" or "What will your grandmother say?"). Keeping giving non-answers until your kid stops talking. If there's genuine trouble afoot, you can deal with it in due time. If you diffuse the initial shock value, the trouble may blow right over. When teenagers try to provoke a reaction, don't give them the satisfaction. Don't react.

. . . .

Practicing the art of detachment while getting to know what's going on with our teenagers takes guts, patience and resilience. Often, it's best to maintain this distance. Other times, it's important to take a more active role in knowing them. We look to another new role model to help us.

Chapter Ten

Ninja
(Disarm Them)

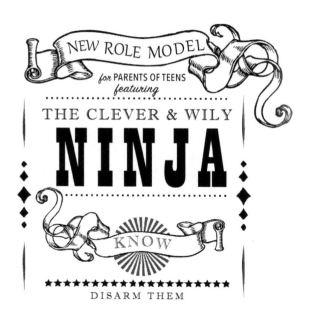

NEW ROLE MODEL

for PARENTS OF TEENS

featuring

THE CLEVER & WILY

NINJA

KNOW

DISARM THEM

ANOTHER CLEVER WAY to know our teenagers is to ambush them, to show up when they least expect us. For this task we look to another new role model, the Ninja: silent, sneaky, prone to appearing out of nowhere. The Ninja can help us disarm teenagers and keep them on their toes, which often leads to knowing them much better and gives us precious glimpses into the lives they are actually leading. Even more to the point, let us recall sometimes-ninja Cato, Inspector Clouseau's karate-chopping manservant in the *Pink Panther* canon. Hired to keep the good inspector vigilant, Cato's stealthy and unexpected attacks underscore the power of surprise. While the parent as Private Investigator lurks in the shadows, the Ninja parent jumps out from the bushes every now and again. As our teenagers seek space, distance, secrecy, privacy and way less time with us, sometimes an unexpected appearance is the only shot we have at knowing what's going on with them. Here, some active things we can do inspired by our new role model the Ninja:

SHOW UP.

Some adolescents happily invite parents to games, concerts and awards ceremonies. They're okay hanging out with friends and family simultaneously. Many others, however, would convince the world they have, in fact, no parents at all. Just lone wolves wandering the suburban streets, these kids. They beg parents to leave them alone. They are humiliated when we're around. They shun us and say nasty things to us and it's tempting to give up on them altogether. We know we can't give up, so like a Ninja, we can show up.

At all the events they beg us not to attend: show up. If your presence truly embarrasses them, move stealthily (like a Ninja). Stand in the shadows. Speak softly. But be there. I know parents who have hung out in parking lots and the outfield during middle school baseball games, snuck into the back row during choir concerts and lurked in shadows during awards banquets. But they were there. I recently met a dad who, when his daughter was in high school, learned which locker was hers. A few times each year he'd drop by while she was in class and leave little notes: "Hi, Honey! Hope you're having a good day! Love, Dad." Brilliant. Can you imagine how unnerved she must have been? Likewise, we can pop in for lunch where they're eating, take walks through parks where they hang out, or go see a movie (which just happens to be showing next to the movie they're seeing. Wave hello; pay for their popcorn; leave them alone). It's the unexpected showing up that counts. The Ninja parent keeps teenagers on their toes.

A certain fundraising office keeps calling me, and I keep recognizing the number and not answering. They have called 15 times in two months. I guess they figure eventually I will break down and give them what they want. Or maybe they think one of these days they'll catch me in the right mood to receive their pleas for cash, and I will cave. Showing up, Ninja-style, takes exactly this brand of tenacity. We have to keep calling. We have to keep showing up, loving them when they push us away (the same children who once needed our snuggles to feel right with the world), smiling at them when they abuse us, telling them they are awesome even when they reject all praise.

And this is important: we might stop praising them when they tell us it's annoying. We might stop showing up at games when everything about us humiliates them. We might stop feeding them when we get sick of hearing the intricacies of how awful our cooking is. We might stop reminding them how to clean the toilet when week after disgusting week their bathroom becomes condemnable—we might want to let them live like street rats and suffer the consequences—and they might never learn how to actually clean up after themselves. As much as they protest, we must keep showing up. The Ninja gets creative and so can parents. We can appear at moments they don't expect, ready and waiting when their mood shifts and they weaken to our efforts. If my husband had stopped telling our son his golf swing was really coming along—a compliment the child rejected for a good four years—he would not have seen the satisfied look on our boy's face when he finally heard it at age 16. If we are good Ninjas who make surprise appearances, we will enjoy moments like these. Our kids will accept a compliment or smile at a joke. They will even show signs of loving us again and we will be connected. But if we are not vigilant and persistent and annoying in our love, if we lose interest or take their abuse personally, if we hibernate or collapse from all the exhaustion, those moments will never come.

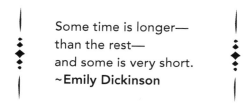

Some time is longer—
than the rest—
and some is very short.
~Emily Dickinson

SPEND TIME WITH THEM: FORCE FAMILY FUN.

Our time with these teenagers is short, though it is endless. We tend to wish away the years until the *doppelgängers* are replaced by our old, familiar, loving progeny. It's awfully difficult to remain engaged with people who are so regularly—so thoroughly, personally and painfully—nasty to you. When our teenagers develop attitudes and start to reject us, it's literally adding insult to injury. Oh, it is so tempting to check out.

We know better. We understand the importance of living in the present. While raising, living with and doing the laundry of our teenagers, we do best to act like we want to be here. To that end, I recommend Forced Family Fun with teenagers. We must keep expectations low; remember, we're essentially hanging out with toddlers, who are not known for their relaxing qualities. Amidst the bickering and *ennui* inspired by these times

102

together, try to find ways to laugh. To make memories. Fleeting moments of joy shared with teenagers are worth the pain of getting there. Give thanks; bank the memory; forget the horrible parts; do it again and again.

Parents, let us act like we want to be here for these few remaining years with our children still in the nest. Let us engage with them so we know who they really are. Let us open our eyes to any real danger so we can protect them on their journey toward adulthood. Let us honor them enough to let them fail; let us always remind them they are worthy of our love. Before we know it—the time is very short—they will be grown and gone. These final years together will be so much sweeter if we try not to wish them away and instead find ways to enjoy them. Keep showing up. Force a little regular family fun. I promise, you won't regret it. Along the way, you'll have the real pleasure of getting to know your kids better.

BREAK BREAD WITH THEM.

If the tyranny of dinner (So much pressure! So much compelling, guilt-inducing evidence in its favor!) sends you over the edge, I am sorry to share this terrible news. The importance of Family Dinner grows right along with our progeny. The upside is that pizza counts.

Parents who know a lot about their teenagers allow great freedom within strict boundaries. They listen more than lecture. They forgive and forget. They cut some slack, but when their kids do truly reprehensible things, these parents get right up in their business. These moms and dads understand the difference between normal teenaged shenanigans and destructive behavior because they know what's going on. How do these parents get so savvy? As always, striking the balance with teens is a daily commitment. The parents I admire face each day with flexibility, tenacity, and a sense of humor. Their secret? There are many, of course, but without exception they insist on the importance of Family Dinner.

Dinner with teenagers is important, despite their chaotic schedules and desire to avoid us. In the homes of parents who know their kids, teens are required to spend time at the table with adults before spending time on their own. Friends are welcome and often present; food is simple and plentiful; hats are removed; dishes are passed with gentility; thanks are given; electronics are *verboten*. Above all, robust conversation is required.

(We also need to admit our limits; dinner together every single night grows more unlikely with more complicated daily itineraries. When we make it a priority and when we celebrate the times it does happen, Family Dinner feels more like a treat and less like torture.)

Three Ways to Get Teenagers to Talk

Here is how clever parents enforce conversation between the generations: they use artificial tactics to structure conversation, they relax their standards and they enjoy each magic moment.

1. Employ Artificial Conversation Tactics.
Several families I know (including mine) stash trivia and conversation-igniting games in the dining room. Clever options abound: Table Topics, Apples to Apples, Cards Against Humanity, even Trivial Pursuit: cards with questions to force conversation in even the most recalcitrant juvenile. Adults must maintain a pedestrian following of the rules (everyone answers; everyone asks a follow-up question) but usually, something ignites curiosity, controversy or comedy. Before you know it, those kids are talking.

Other ploys abound, of course. Some of our impromptu favorites require everyone at the table to:

- tell a joke
- give thanks for one thing
- answer a "would you rather" premise
- make a prediction about the next decade
- describe a favorite childhood lunch
- name the best and worst part of the day
- decide where on their body they would place an extra nose

It is best to keep things light and to forgive kids for squirming and being silly; remember, if they're talking, you're winning.

2. Relax Your Standards. Listen. Let them talk.

Once they start chattering, we've got to relax our standards. Within the boundaries of civilized manners, allow teens at the dinner table to converse like the adolescents they are. Organic conversation happens when we hang back and let teenagers give voice to all the weird expressions of their hormone-infused brain boxes. Here, among the pizza and the Chipotle burritos, is often all the intel we need. Listening to their rambling conversations is a great way to know, protect and honor our almost grown children. They will tell us what they think is funny, what disgusts them, whom they mistrust and whom they long to be.

When they talk, teenagers express unoriginal, incorrect and mis-guided ideas with the conviction of dictators. Within reason and within your family's sense of propriety, let them express themselves without correction or judgment. We, the adults, know their ideas are not unique. We know their comedy is (by definition) juvenile. Let them laugh. Let yourself laugh with them. Let them express their goofiness without shutting them down or minimizing them. Then make them help with the dishes and send them into another room so you can enjoy more intelligent, adult conversation.

3. Don't Ruin the Magic.

We know teenagers tend to communicate at inconvenient times. When we are exhausted, on the phone with the doctor, or rushing to meet a deadline, our kids get talkative.

If you hear yourself saying, "Not now . . . " to your adolescent son or daughter, STOP. Take a breath. Drop what you are doing. Ask your careening-toward-empty-nesting self, "If not now, when?"

If your teen should ask or say something demanding your attention, sit frozen if you must. Ignore hunger, bladder, errands that need running and bedtimes if you are lucky enough to find yourself in the midst of a real conversation. It's like coaxing a squirrel to eat from your hand. You don't want to make any sudden movements or break the magic of the moment.

And what magic it is when teenaged people start spilling their guts! When that veil lifts, amidst their ramblings (if we are patient enough) we will hear secrets, code words, gossip about friends, and the true longings of their confused little hearts. If we pay especially close attention, as their frontal lobes gradually develop, we will hear the whispers of understanding, forgiveness, and even burgeoning, adult respect for us. And then the veil falls and they're grumpy and reticent again. So it is: ephemera, a moment in time, gone just as quickly as it appeared. Magic.

Even as we schedule more formal attempts to get kids to talk, let us not miss their casual, spontaneous, serendipitous (often just so inconvenient!) moments of communication. These unplanned, catch-em-while-you-can moments of conversation reveal the everyday magic of living with teenagers. Our errands can wait; our plans can be rescheduled; our children will never be this age again. Let us seize those fleeting moments of genuine connection when they appear before our very eyes.

. . . .

LET THEM KNOW YOU GET IT.

Parents—like Ninjas—can disarm our teenagers with a line from a popular meme or movie and gain mountains of credibility. Knowing pop culture and contemporary slang is a secret weapon when raising teenagers. You can throw them off their game (thanks to all your research as Private Investigator) when you know what they're talking about. You'll see it happen: they look up startled from their collective slouch like, "What? She knows *that*?" It astonishes them and makes them wonder what else you know. Powerful stuff.

I used this tactic to great advantage when I taught high school. My students hated me at first because I was tough, but they quickly thought I was kinda cool (because I have an adolescent personality and I like the same comedians they like). They tended to trust me. They tended to think I was their friend. Sometimes they revealed more to me than they did their parents and before I knew it, I gained solid intel on all sorts of scary situations. I have an unnaturally high tolerance for teenaged mischief, but when I learn about teenagers in real and present danger, lucky for them, I am not cool and I am not their friend. I used this intelligence against them every time when it came to keeping kids safe. (More on what protecting them looks like from role models in future chapters.)

The teenage ambush takes many forms, of course, including being in unexpected places and staging hand checks in basements full of mixed company. There is one element of surprise, however, parents tend to overlook. And it's the best one, because it can be so much fun.

SHOW THEM YOUR HIDDEN TALENTS.

I have seen it again and again: parents I admire shock the heck out of their adolescent children simply by being themselves. Remember, adolescents are convinced their parents are obsolete, out of date, irrelevant . . . barely even human. It is therefore worth pulling out all the stops, now and again, if just for the sheer pleasure of seeing their jaws drop. (Also, this kind of ambush builds their respect for us.)

Beleaguered parents tend to let certain parts of our personalities fall away. Who has time for all those hobbies and pursuits which made our twenties so interesting? Well, I'm here to tell you, your children' adolescent years are the perfect time to unearth these former passions. [Important Note: there is a difference between showing off in real time and reminiscing, Uncle-Rico-style, about past glories. The former is awesome, the latter often seems pathetic to teenagers.]

. . . .

Nine Ways to Ambush Teens with Your Own Awesomeness

(Some of my favorite examples from parents and teenagers I've interviewed)

1. While traveling with the family in Morocco, Dad recalls enough college-level French to get directions for the whole crew. His progeny are stunned; they didn't know he had ever studied French!

2. A mom with boys—a former athlete who has been mostly sedentary for 12 years—whips out 50 pushups and walks on her hands. The kids are gob smacked.

3. A father (with a Belushi-like physique) silences a pool party with a series of expertly executed back flips and belly flops.

4. A stay-at-home mom returns to her love of pottery and expertly throws mugs, vases and bowls on the wheel, a skill not lost on her high school kids, struggling in ceramics class. (This mom was me!)

5. A working woman with sons—who have never paid a bit of attention to her J-O-B—announces one night at dinner she is, at last, prepared to buy her company. And then she does. The boys eventually write their essays for admission to business school about it.

6. A guy with a bit of a public persona is invited to join a cow-milking competition to celebrate the opening of a new local business. His 13-year-old kid, certain of the resulting humiliation, is shocked instead: seems his daddy grew up on a farm, and milking is like riding a bike. He wins the crazy contest; the kid is relieved and strangely proud.

7. A blue-collar dad, rarely seen without his ball cap and untucked shirt, cleans up beautifully for a father-daughter dance and

109

remembers enough moves from cotillion to make his girl feel like a princess on the dance floor.

8. On a family car ride, a radio station announces a best impression contest and Mom calls in with her spot-on sendup of Keith Richards, which the children have never heard. Dad is not surprised when she wins the cash prize; the impersonation was one of the reasons he loved her in the first place.

9. A family of five nearly grown children relishes the moment when each new kid is introduced to Mom and Dad's Dirty Dancing lift scene "...or the 'run and jump,' as we call it," their daughter writes. (These are such socially responsible and always appropriate parents, the image is all the more delightful.)

. . . .

Parents, don't hide your light under a bushel! Let it shine. Illuminate the cobwebby corners of your real personality and show your teenagers just some of the clever, crazy, cool things you can do. They may never quite recover . . and you can use their bewilderment to reconnect with them during these awful, awkward years. Shine on!

Parents who know their teens can take steps to protect and honor them, as well. When—and only when—our kids are in real and present danger, what must we do to swoop in and protect them? Remember: every child, every situation is different. We walk a fine line. Protecting our children can take many forms. Our new role models, beyond Mama Bear and all her hibernating, can help us.

ROLE MODELS
WHO PROTECT

THE SOLDIER
THE TREE
THE ENGLISH TEACHER
THE PERSONAL TRAINER
THE PRESCHOOL TEACHER

Chapter Eleven

Soldier
(Guard Them)

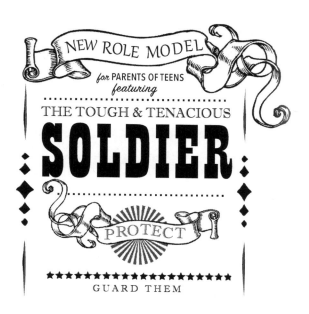

SECURE THE PERIMETERS.

If teenagers are like toddlers (and they are), they need help remembering their boundaries. A 14-year-old, much like a three-year-old, needs to be reminded about basic cause-and-effect phenomena. The stove is hot! The street is dangerous! Laundry in the basket gets washed; clothing on the floor does not! Homework turned into the teacher gets graded; homework left in your backpack does not! Toddlers, however, are adorable and relatively easy to placate. With teenagers, stakes are higher and the danger is real. As the experts tell us, teenagers are in peril because they are programmed to do peculiar, rash things. Teens are biologically commanded to rebel, to test limits, to seek danger. Parents need to actively reinforce their boundaries, in equal measure to how actively the teens transgress and push limits. As we leave Mama Bear, then, to her hibernation, let us look to the Soldier for inspiration.

On a recent visit to New York City, I was aware of the silent but powerful presence of armed military guards in Grand Central Station. They said nothing; they appeared intimidating and approachable all at once; I felt safer because they were there. I didn't feel threatened but I sure felt watched. I was aware of my movements and manners. Above all, there was a subtle reassurance that if any screwy stuff should hit the fan, there in the vast sea of anonymous humanity, someone would be there to make it all right.

That, My Friends, is the kind of parent we often need to be. The Soldier sacrifices personal comfort and convenience in service of a greater good (such as raising our children to responsible adulthood). Soldiers have to be strong and do their jobs, even in inhumane conditions. They take endless abuse, swallow their pride, remain loyal beyond reason, and never, never, never rest when the battle is raging. All of which is not unlike parenting teenagers. Good things are worth fighting for; our kids are worth it. Parenting like a Soldier means reinforcing and patrolling the borders to keep camp safe. We decide what boundaries we will hold for our kids—they are different for every family—and we secure our perimeters. Although I have very strong opinions on things like sex and drugs and drinking and schoolwork, each family must draw the boundaries we think are appropriate to keep our families safe and healthy. And then we protect those boundaries with everything we've got.

Lest we worry about the militant images this role model conjures, let me remind you we're playing a part. Like all our new role models, the Soldier is a hat we put on only when necessary. The life of a teenager is messy and complicated and hormonal. Our kids are under pressures we may not understand and they can't fully be trusted to set good boundaries for themselves (because of those highly susceptible adolescent brains). Parenting like a Soldier means scaffolding the decision-making process for them. Teenagers are compelled to rebel and push limits. If they have no limits to test, they face the void of existence on their own before they are mature enough to do so. So we help them. We accept our role as the face of authority, of rules, of order and good sense. When they reject boundaries but need them to stay safe, our teenagers can blame us. We give shape to their limits; we are the voice that says "no." The reason I look to the Soldier for inspiration is because it's a demanding job, protecting people who so actively, passionately reject boundaries. Soldiers face life-or-death decisions every day. Often, so do teenagers (and their parents). Let us be tough as Soldiers and strong enough to take whatever nasty things our kids do as part of their rebellion.

Eight Ways to Protect Teenagers like a Soldier

1. Giving consequences for breaking rules: We may have to set curfews and other rules that are unpopular with our children and their friends.

2. Having awkward conversations: Well, we have decided that smoking weed is not okay for a 14-year-old, but we know there's a lot of pressure to do so. So we will be giving pee tests at home, and you can tell everyone you can't indulge because of your horrible parents. Please blame us.

3. Being the heavy: Protecting may mean confiscating video games and cell phones and even the car. It certainly means tearful, angry arguments and ugly, rebellious behavior. It may mean taking abuse and suffering insults (because everyone else is going. Because you are so unreasonable and so insensitive). Remember: the shape of their rebellion takes the shape of your soul. It gets personal. Teenagers denied their privileges (technology, vehicles, social lives) act not unlike inmates during a riot. You have the protective gear of perspective, because you are not a teenager. You have the armor of adulthood. Sometimes, it helps to visualize yourself strapping on shield and sword. Channel whatever source of strength you have. You can take it, parents; Soldier on!

4. Fetching teenagers from bad places: It might mean staying sober, awake, and dressed until midnight so you can pick your child up from a party where boys and girls are spending the night together (which is happening with alarming frequency in our circle—whaaaat?).

5. Making phone calls: to their friends or their friends' parents or their teachers or coaches.

6. Yelling at strangers: who offer your kid drugs or who make inappropriate comments or gestures (remember yelling at strangers who drove down your block too fast when toddlers were playing in the front yard? Same deal).

7. Monitoring their online activity (I hope this goes without saying): knowing passwords, aliases, ghost accounts; staying one step ahead of them on the computers; setting up accounts to read their texts and snap chats; limiting video-game time, which can become a serious addiction in high school and college, as damaging as a drug addiction.

8. Spending a day back in high school: Oh, boy, I love this one. Certain parents of wayward youth arrange to accompany the little hooligan to a full day of school. They promise to sit quietly in the back of the room, just to observe, to get an accurate perspective, don't you know. [Hint: only once did this beautiful proposition come to fruition in my classroom. The real threat—time taken off from work, honest availability and willingness on behalf of the parent—in every other case was enough to change the problem behavior, and fast. Brilliant.]

BOUNDARIES ARE BEAUTIFUL.

Every day in a million ways, adolescents will show us how much they hate the very boundaries they need to feel okay with the world. Stay strong, parents. Without rules, boundaries and some sense of order, the world gets tumultuous for teenagers. When they get away with too much nonsense, they unintentionally get the upper hand and lose respect for our authority. They see us as the weak, vulnerable human beings we really are, which can be confounding and scary for them. (In good time, of course, they'll learn to see us as imperfect people doing our best. But during these years of hormonal formation, they are not quite ready for that kind of truth.) Until their frontal lobes fully form and they are capable of making rational, long-term decisions for themselves, they need us to help do it for them. So let us take comfort in knowing we give them what they need, rather than what they think they want. For more inspiration when they test our limits in creative, personal, painful ways, let's look to other role models who help us protect our teenagers.

Chapter Twelve

Tree
(Shelter Them)

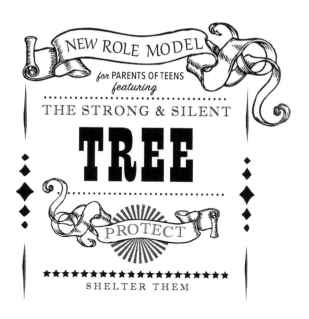

ON A RECENT country drive, I was struck by the graceful shelterbelts standing at attention throughout the fields in precise, military rows. If you have motored across rural America, you've seen these regular outcrop-pings of trees: straight, stately columns in the low-slung expanse of prairie.

These trees serve many purposes: wind reduction, snow protection, wild-life habitat and reducing soil erosion. Good farmers take shelterbelts seriously, knowing they protect precious topsoil as well as family and livestock. Children raised in the country, however, tend to see shel-terbelts in a more enchanted light. Unlike the dark, sprawling, scary forests of fairy tales and fables, shelterbelts are planned and planted by human hands, shelter indeed because they are knowable. They are small, contained, safe. In a shelterbelt, farm kids feel at home but in the wild at once: free to test limits, explore the nature of things and move amidst wild beasts, knowing all the while safety and shelter are just a field away. A shelterbelt provides freedom within boundaries and an environment in which to commune with the essence of life. Pretty much everything I hope to do for my almost adult children.

In the wild privacy of shelterbelts, kids build tree houses and forts. They escape summer heat on the cool, pine-duff forest floor and carve tunnels into massive snow drifts forced between tree trunks by winter winds. They collect vacated nests, play hide-and-seek and steal first kisses. If they hunt, they seek relative shelter in the frozen hour before dawn and wait. If they love the company of bunnies and other woodland creatures, they hunt only with soft voices, gifts of carrots or insects, and imaginary play. (When the man I love best was himself a teenager, he sat breathless in a shelterbelt while his older brother scared a herd of mule deer into the trees. He recalls the thrill of sitting undetected among 100 nervous, truly wild animals. As he raised his bow and arrow, he grazed a branch; the deer scattered; he didn't get a shot. But the moment profoundly moved him.)

Like these hard-working trees, parents need to stand tall against the storms of adolescence. We are rooted in experience and tough enough to bend with the punishing winds. And so here, in an homage to my own rural upbringing, five reasons parenting teenagers means planting and maintaining a shelterbelt.

Five Things a Tree Taught Me about Parenting

1. A parent's job is to stand there. Engaging with teens is often ugly, complicated, and bound for argument. We should keep seeking communication with them, of course, but sometimes it really is best to just be there. In the next room, when they call, when they get chatty, when their anger is misplaced squarely at us. When we feel like running away and joining the circus. Just stand there. You can take it. You're a tree.

2. Parents are visible boundaries. Columns of trees trace property lines, riverbeds, and rural roads, serving as guideposts and borders. Much like parents of teenagers. Never forget the power of your presence.

3. When you walk among giant trees, you get the feeling they've seen everything. They're old. They seem somehow wise in their silent, noble photosynthesis: just breathing to the ancient rhythms of the planet while we scurry and worry below. Like silent elders. Like parents. Trust your ability to have an effect on your children even when they seem impenetrable. Laugh gently and knowingly as the adolescent drama shakes your branches. Let the little miscreants carve their initials into your hearty trunk. Smile patiently. It's just a scratch; it's nothing; they can't really harm you. You're a tree.

121

4. Parents, like trees, need sunlight, water and nutrients. Take care of yourself. You know what you need to do to stay healthy; try to do it all, as much as your zany schedule will allow. Keep a clear head and remember the beating of your own heart, which is often all you've got. Take care of yourself.

5. Trees and parents spread deep, wide roots. Every graceful, upright tree sends a tangle of shoots and suckers in an underground search for nourishment. Likewise, conversations with parents of friends, teachers, or mentors keep us connected to our willful, rebellious progeny. The traditions, rituals and manners we enforce—going to church despite epic resistance, spending time with curmudgeonly grandparents, writing thank you notes—also grow like roots, right into the developing character of our children. Hang in there; stay vigilant; trust your influence. Reach out and spread roots when you need your community to step in and help you.

Chapter Thirteen

English Teacher
(Equip Them)

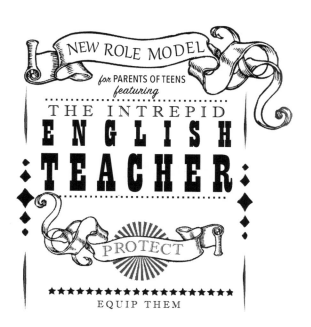

WHY DID I TEACH GRAMMAR TO KIDS WHO HATED IT?

We do not like to admit it, but parents cannot truly keep our kids safe. The storms threaten with too much force; the best we can do is offer some shelter. The best protection is knowing how to think. Messages from corporations, institutions and industries barrage our kids every minute of every day. The only real shelter lies within themselves: the ability to discern good from bad, right from wrong, and truth from deceit. This is the key to ultimate, adult liberty: being free to make choices unfettered by ignorance. This is also why I endeavored to teach high school English. It's also why the English Teacher is an important role model for those of us trying to protect our teenagers.

RHETORIC IS POWER.

Although some students remember me fondly, I was not the kind of teacher who inspired a lifelong romance with literature. As I reminded them often, I didn't give a whit how much they liked a book (only I didn't say "whit"). We had bigger fish to fry. Namely, I wanted my students to graduate with a solid command of language and rhetoric. I wanted to see improvement in their ability to make and deconstruct an argument. More specifically, I wanted to strengthen their bullshit detectors so they would have shelter against the arguments preying constantly upon their beautiful brains.

Most high school students would rather talk about anything besides grammar. Literary analysis interests them only slightly more. Discussions of tone, theme, purpose—and Heaven forbid syntax or diction—inspire resentment, apathy, even violence in the average teenager. And yet, nearly every day of my teaching career, I insisted on talking about grammar and analysis. And it was awful. I didn't care how deeply the *Twilight* series moved them personally; I wanted to know if they could protect themselves from the barrage of arguments aimed at them 24/7. It was drills, diagrams and repetitive, scaffolded exercises. All. Day. Long. They hated me. They wanted to bring me down. Why not change tack? Why make it so rough for myself and unpleasant for them? Why sail against rough winds instead of taking the smoother course of young-adult lit and how it makes kids feel? Because their brains are worth it. Because, by Jove, they became better writers and readers because of it. Maybe they'll know when a politician or advertiser or newscaster is selling them down the river with a logical fallacy.

Adults have the opportunity (if not the mandate) to teach kids how to protect their brains against predators. In our brave new world of constant media messaging, the task is more vital than ever. I lost sleep over teenagers who fought my instruction (due to their unfortunate, adolescent circumstances) because unless we understand how arguments work, we are powerless against the arguments invading our mind-grapes.

CRITICAL MINDS BUILD STRONG BACKBONES.

These almost adults will soon be making decisions about where they spend their money, whom they support in elections, and how they conduct themselves in the wide, weird world. Our parental, teaching, and grown up decree is to give them shelter from the storms threatening to blow them off course.

So we diagram sentences. We learn the rules of syntax. We write formulaically in the classroom until we can prove a thesis with airtight precision. It's brutal work, but the minds of our future adults are worth the struggle. When they know how to defend a logical argument of their own (which begins with knowing how to craft a smart sentence), students are more capable of recognizing the fallacies in the arguments aimed squarely at them.

125

The forces threatening our teenagers (and all of us) are too many to fathom. Nary a parent I know would argue against the importance of fortifying our children's inner strength in the face of all the evils in the world. That strength—that ability to make sound, responsible decisions—begins and ends with understanding the messages we receive and interpreting them wisely.

Let us give our teenagers the shelter of strong backbones and critical minds. The study of rhetoric, which begins with grammar and embraces logical argument, is an excellent place to start.

See you in English class.

. . . .

Five Ways to Parent like an English Teacher:

1. Language is a Tool: Use It.

This is my particular weakness. I am infamous for insisting on proper grammar and punctuation. More importantly, though, I try to convince teenagers they can wield the power of words to their advantage. We are all writers, I promise them, who rely on good communication to shape our lives. Whether we are applying for jobs, organizing people, raising funds for good causes, running for office or trying to get along with our spouses, we do best to respect the power of language. The English Teacher role model instructs us to be specific and precise as we communicate our wants and needs, our opinions and our positions. A carpenter would never use a hammer on a Philips-head screw. English Teachers give students a tool box of syntax, vocabulary and the power to use those tools well. Parents can channel this role model by rejecting vague responses to questions, teaching our kids "big words" and how to use them precisely, and requiring them to make sense of their sometimes nonsensical adolescent gibberish.

2. Cite Your Sources.

While it is perfectly natural, normal and necessary for teenagers to mimic ideas, hairstyles and attitudes, the English Teacher role model reminds them that plagiarism is forbidden. The ultimate goal is to help our children define and assert their own ideas. We are grateful for any input—from philosophers to pop bands to reality shows—that informs their world view. But we are also careful to help them distinguish between the forces at work on their psyches and their own beliefs and passions. Parents can challenge our teenagers to acknowledge their inspirations rather than steal from them. We can assist their development as human beings by teaching them to be part of the great, cosmic conversation, wherein we learn from one another as we establish our own unique identities.

3. Give Good Evidence.

Adolescents make some wild claims. They tend to believe dramatic rumors and draw hysterical conclusions. A good English Teacher suffers no such nonsense. "Provide evidence," we cry, and we teach them how to do it. The same is true for parents: we can protect our teenagers from the raging winds of misinformed opinion by reminding them to present data or other proof to support whatever they believe. We can ask them to explore their underlying assumptions and to explain (or analyze) their beliefs. It can feel a bit like coaching our own family debate team. As far as this English Teacher is concerned, that's a good thing. Rational, logical rhetoric is the stuff that dreams are made on. Without it, we fall victim to the media and other sinister stimuli.

4. Always Be Skeptical; Never Get Cynical

Teaching high school students to "be skeptical" was one of my favorite parts of teaching. Questioning authority is right in their wheelhouse; they do it naturally and often inappropriately. We can use this tendency to help them seek logic and rationality. When they recognize hypocrisy or inconsistency, when they suspect someone is lying or glossing over the truth, we can encourage teenagers to get to the bottom of things. Once again, the English Teacher role model reminds us to make them do research, cite sources and find the fallacies in any argument. The English Teacher, however, also believes in the power of literature and entertainment to save our souls. Even the darkest authors write to bring some glimmer of hope to the human condition. Writers across time buck traditions, ask difficult questions and challenge boundaries, much like teenagers do. But ultimately they help us make sense of things. They write, in fact, to keep from getting cynical. Our English Teacher role model is especially valuable as we steer kids away from pessimism and contempt. We believe our children can get better as long as they don't get bitter.

Many, many men have been just as troubled morally and spiritually as you are right now. Happily, some of them kept records of their troubles. You'll learn from them—if you want to. Just as someday, if you have something to offer, someone will learn something from you. It's a beautiful reciprocal arrangement. And it isn't education. It's history. It's poetry.
~J.D. Salinger, *The Catcher in the Rye* (Mr. Antolini)

5. Just Say It.
Good teachers of every subject know the trick we call economy of language. When giving instructions, it's best to speak clearly and concisely and then shut up. Explaining things five different ways at once is too much for students—especially teenagers—to absorb. They receive information best in small, digestible chunks. When adolescent drama arises (and it will), parents retain the important

upper hand by using economy of language. Teenagers in trouble tend to blabber and tell half-truths and get mired in trivial details. Parenting like an English Teacher means we say what we need to say; we get the information we need; we explain consequences clearly and concisely; we shut up. It's a powerful method, because often a teenager—fueled by hormones and itching for a fight—wants to wallow in a long, emotional *tête-à-tête*. These conversations are almost always fruitless, pointless and exhausting. When parents remain detached and use fewer actual words in our communication, we put a swifter end to the nonsense. Craft your message with care; lay it on them; drop your microphone and get off the stage.

Parenting Mic Drop
ˈpʰerˑənˑtɪŋ ˈmaɪk ˈdrɑp

1. An instance of deliberately dropping or tossing aside one's (imaginary) microphone at the end of a speech one considers to have landed with particular impact on one's audience of recalcitrant teenagers.

'she made her point with a parenting mic drop after announcing there would be no screen time for two weeks, end of story.'

1.1 [as exclamation] Used to emphasize that a discussion is at an end after a definitive or particularly impressive point has been made.

'Nuff said. Your rooms need to be clean by 5:00. Mic drop.'

Chapter Fourteen

Personal Trainer
(Work Them)

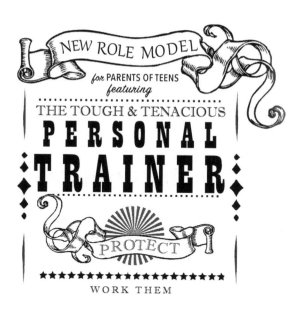

AS WE KNOW, the adolescent brain is an open window, vulnerable and susceptible to all outside influences. We also know the active re-wiring taking place during these years—designed to prepare our kids for adulthood—is a great opportunity. Teenagers are receptive to everything: positive as well as negative influences. We take best advantage of this phenomenon (and protect our kids from danger) by turning up the positive, turning down the negative and teaching them to practice healthy habits.

Like so many interactions with teens, getting them to exercise, eat well and stay disciplined can be maddening. Teenagers crave idleness but building healthy bodies takes so much work! Scaffolding healthy routines and daily habits for them feels like so much maintenance! And it is. Our homes, vehicles, relationships, careers and bodies must be tended to constantly, daily, consistently. Maintenance is a form of protection: against weather, age, apathy, obsolescence, and any other indignities the world might throw our way. But maintenance is difficult, even for most successful adults. It takes serious discipline. One of the women I look up to the most in all the world, who seems wise and put together, as if she knows the secret to life, reminded me what a struggle it is to make good, healthy choices each day. "I know everything in my day will go better if I eat protein for breakfast and take a morning walk. I know it! But every single day I want to eat crackers and do a crossword puzzle at the kitchen table! Every. Single. Day." We feel her pain, don't we?

It's hard. We seek all kinds of inspiration: calendars and scheduling apps, support groups and benevolent friends, professional therapy, yoga and spinning classes. Sometimes in the name of fitness, we hire a trainer to keep us on track. Let us turn, then, to the Personal Trainer to help us help our teenagers. Here is a role model of consistency, discipline and positive encouragement, who embodies the importance of repetition, of skills and drills and working hard for good results. To protect teenagers, sometimes parents need to work them. Whether it means insisting upon regular physical exercise, daily chores or real jobs, let us look to the Personal Trainer when our teenagers need this kind of protection. When we know what's going on and we determine our children need us to protect them from laziness, apathy, raging hormones, chaos, low self-esteem, disease, boredom, self pity or inertia, the Personal Trainer instructs us.

MAKE THEM WORK OUT.

All of us need exercise. We know it, and we know myriad reasons why. One reason is because it keeps us sane; it helps us keep our challenges in perspective. We think better, sleep better and feel better when we engage in regular exercise (no matter how much we resist it). All these benefits are especially important for teenagers and the aggressive, hormonal chemistry percolating in their grey matter. If your adolescent children play sports or get other regular exercise, you may be in the clear on this one. If, however, your kids tend toward inactivity (or video games, Netflix binges or other sedentary pursuits) you may have to play the part of Personal Trainer and get them off the couch.

Physical exercise—even a daily walk—can help protect our teenagers from hormonal surges, sloth and poor general health. In the gym, trainers maintain positive attitudes, shout encouraging words from the sidelines and put us through our paces even when we don't feel like doing anything. The parent as Personal Trainer does the same. As it is with so much of parenting, this role can be exhausting and we may meet great resistance. We must channel our indefatigable new role model and try to meet every complaint with cheerful insistence. If we sense our kids need more exercise, we might organize family hikes or kickball games. We might have to sacrifice our own longing for lazy weekend mornings and insist on walking with our kids. Or swimming, skiing, boxing, paddle boarding, canoeing or hot yoga classes. You catch my drift. When teenagers get lost, we cannot underestimate their need for physical activity: stress-relieving, hormone-releasing, brain-balancing, good-for-your-body exercise. I'm leaning heavily on observation here but I'm pretty sure science backs me up: to function at their best and overcome their unfortunate, adolescent condition, teenagers need to break a sweat every single day.

I am in awe of one intrepid mother who runs three times a week with her daughter. But get this: because the sweet young thing hates to be seen in public with her mom, they run different routes. They drive together to a neighborhood trail, run in opposite directions and meet back at the car for a slightly less sullen ride home. I am humbled by my friend's tenacity and commitment to parenting. Even though the circumstances are less than perfect, she insists on their running time together and makes the very best of it. Both of them benefit (and I have a hunch one of these days, when the daughter's brain is more mature, she'll agree to run alongside her mother again).

In the most recalcitrant teenagers, exercise may be a way to earn screen time or other less active privileges. Here again, it's an exhausting job, but the parent as Personal Trainer might design—and enforce—programs of sacrifice and reward. Most of the time I prefer a hands-off, face-your-own-consequences parenting style, but being firm (and authoritative) sometimes means a lot of nagging. It can mean charts hanging on the refrigerator, using technology as currency, and diplomatic-level negotiations. Like the Personal Trainer who creates workout schedules and diet plans, our real job is to make sure the plans are followed, which takes daily attention and constant maintenance, neither of which teenagers are usually able to do fully on their own. Eventually, we trust, these skills we nourish and tend will flourish into sound reasoning and good decision making. By scaffolding their ability to delay gratification (screen time or lazy afternoons), we help them mature into responsible and capable adults.

Authoritative parents have high expectations for their children and give them the resources and support they need to succeed. Exercise can be just such a resource for many teenagers. Sloth, inertia and hormones are a poisonous combination, usually resulting in pent-up frustrations and odd, uncontrollable outbursts. Sometimes teenagers make terrible, desperate decisions despite themselves and what they know is right. In these situations, when they need some correction or consequences, experience shows me that hard, physical work can make a world of difference. Active chores around the house can serve both parents and wayward teens: they may scrub baseboards or wash windows, clean gutters or move heavy furniture, all in the name of exorcising—and exercising—their adolescent demons. My experience also tells me (I know this is strangely specific) that a couple hours shoveling rock, preferably on a hot summer's day, can transform anger and attitude into peace and calm. I've seen it happen again and again. A young lad who has done something stupid, who perhaps needs a little correction, becomes as gentle as a lamb after two hours of shoveling rock. I have considered installing a big pile of gravel and a wheelbarrow in our backyard, to be perpetually moved back and forth whenever our boys need an outlet for their angst or a consequence for their misdeeds. More practically, I suggest parents have a ready list of friends, neighbors or charities in need of help with yardwork, snow shoveling or trash pick-up. Hard work and service can alter their brain chemistry and their perspective while giving them time to think about their transgressions. Something else for you to try today!

Parenting like a Personal Trainer is most helpful and appropriate when parents need to protect our vulnerable teenagers from the predators of laziness, bad habits and poor health. We can, furthermore, protect them from feeling entitled, living in a fantasy world, shirking responsibility and not understanding how life works. Sometimes, parenting in this fashion means insisting on real exercise and physical work. Sometimes, it means helping them learn how to work, like at an actual job.

MAKE THEM WORK REAL JOBS.

The parent as Personal Trainer cheerfully and relentlessly enforces daily habits that scaffold responsibility. We might feel like giant nags, reminding them to pick up their socks, do their homework, pack their lunches or close cupboard doors. But the Personal Trainer knows it's all part of making them better, more fit for adulthood, so we coach them through their work without resentment, like it's our job (because it is our job). Working as part of the family means carrying our weight, doing chores for communal benefit, and taking responsibility for our own actions and messes. Parents as Personal Trainers scaffold this process and gradually transition kids into real, paid jobs.

Paid work teaches teenagers how to be accountable, persistent and confident in new situations. Work develops good manners, builds understanding of money management and helps young people set priorities and stay organized. The parents I admire require their teenagers to hold jobs, even kids who are varsity athletes and super-students who look forward to full-ride scholarships. Even kids who juggle activities and service projects and volunteer positions. These kids hold jobs as much as makes sense: in the summer months, on weekends, a few evening hours a week. The parents help their daughters and sons with the process of finding their first employment. It can be a scary process, applying for a job out there in the real world! Parents can be like Personal Trainers and help with applications and résumés, as much as our kids will allow. We can help them get training or make contacts for jobs that interest them (babysitting or lifeguard courses, an introduction to our friend who needs help with a summer construction project). We can boost their confidence and make sure they dress appropriately for their interviews. When they are younger, we can drive them to and from work (or help them figure out the bus schedule). Like satisfied Personal Trainers, we will witness the transformation of our teenagers. Before our eyes, they will become more self-assured, more confident in their abilities, and proud of their first tastes of financial independence. Soon enough, they will be able to find and hold jobs on their own. I'm not advocating for child labor, mind you, but the teenagers I know who have real jobs tend to gain a better perspective on their lives. They are less prone to petty drama when they understand the value of hard work.

IT'S A FINE LINE.

Some parents worry, "But they have the rest of their lives to work! They're only young for a short time! Shouldn't these years be for play?" My first answer is, "No they need to work. Work is a way for parents to protect teenagers from a host of dangers." My second and simultaneous answer, however, is, "Yes! A thousand times, yes! Teenagers need to play!" They also need to rest and enjoy downtime. Here we are again at the crux of our struggle: it's a fine, fine line.

Remember: there is no one answer, no rule book, no manual and very little consistency. Remember: step back from the pandemonium and ask, "Do I know what's going on? Must I step in to protect my child from real and present danger? Can I honor my child's unique and imperfect journey toward adulthood?" Only when we know what is truly happening with each kid can we determine our course of action. Only then can we decide what we must do to protect them and honor them. It may look different every single time.

Often, we believe it best to make our teenagers finish what they've started. We channel the Soldier who enforces boundaries and the Personal Trainer who gives constant, positive support, and we help them stay their course, believing lessons learned in the end will be worth it. Other times, we become convinced it's best to let our child quit. When an activity, class, or task is making them truly suffer, when their self-esteem is at stake or they are being abused or mistreated, we cut them some slack and help them get out of a bad situation. We're forever walking that tightrope, seeking balance amidst all the crazy clowns. Step right up and see the death-defying feat of parenting teenagers!

And so, Dear Reader, I will now beg you to use caution when protecting teenagers. Here is a caveat to be judicious always, lest we helicopter, force solutions or micromanage their lives. I am now going to try to convince you that just as often as we need to guard them, shelter them, equip them and work them, we need to chill way out and let them be. Next, I'll introduce you to some role models who guide us toward this balance.

PARENTING CASE STUDY:
Hiking as Family Philosophy

Growing up, mine was a hiking family. When we vacationed and relocated (we moved a lot) to new parts of the country—from tropical forests to lush woods to barren deserts—we got to know our surroundings on foot. My intrepid parents filled water bottles and backpacks and led my siblings and me (through various stages of willingness, apathy and downright resentment) up and down mountain paths and historical trails, encouraging us to know local flora and fauna and hints of human progress.

As small children we loved investigating tracks and trail scat; sensing wildlife so close exhilarated us. We checked seasonal blooms in our wildflower guides (an acceptable excuse to take breaks when the elevation got the better of us. Also a handy tactic for grabbing a snack). We learned rudimentary survival skills and the art of minimal impact: we took only photos and left only footprints. We thrilled at signs of new life in fragile ecosystems and memorized the calls of coyotes, marmots and distant hawks. We respected the violent whims of Mother Nature, equating the smell of ozone above tree line with impending lightning, recognizing the dizzying signs of altitude sickness, digging trenches to protect campsites during flash floods. We developed expert opinions on—and world-class recipes for—trail mix. We read maps. We knew it was cheesy (especially as we explored the fourteeners and ghost towns of Colorado) but we sang John Denver songs with wild abandon whenever we got a chance.

Hard Work + Physical Pain = Nicer Teenagers

Even the specter of adolescence couldn't ruin the lessons of hiking. My teenaged siblings and I—along with the friends our parents begrudgingly let us bring along—woke before daylight with less enthusiasm (and more grumbling profanities) than we once had. We made nasty comments, wielded surly attitudes and generally made a mockery of the proceedings as long as we could. But the reality of physical exertion, along with the undeniable force of natural beauty, got the better of us every time. Now, in my own middle age, with my own teenagers hell-bent on destroying any attempt at family fun, I am amazed at my mom and dad's abject patience.

I know we rolled our eyes at the adults when they complained it was so much worse coming down a mountain. As we young people, invigorated and light-headed from the summit, leaped and tumbled down, our pathetic parents complained of aching knees and wounded hips. It took me until my middle forties to understand, and the knee pain on an easy descent came with a humbling vengeance. What a drag it is getting old. Here is one secret of raising a family my parents understood: the more exhausted teenagers are from hard work, the more likely they are to crash at a reasonable hour, stay out of trouble and leave you to yourselves. Brilliant. While my friends attended weekend keggers, on hiking days I was more inclined to soak blisters in Epsom salts at the kitchen table and make solid plans to get to bed.

The hikes we took with our family, no matter how reluctantly we participated, formed the best parts of my siblings and me. We are people who believe we can survive, in the wilderness or a new job or a city we've never seen before. We know the value of being prepared but we can improvise like nobody's business, no matter where life takes us. There's wilderness and there's urban wilderness. Turns out we were trained pretty well for both.

Markers on the Trail: You Are Here

One thing I loved about hiking with my family and friends, no matter how tired, grumpy or out-of-shape I might have been, was the presence of cairns along the trails. Although I was never truly lost with my parents at the helm, when my adolescent friends and I set out on various adventures we tended to lose our way. How often cairns—those lovingly stacked piles of stones, left by unknown and unseen adventurers before us—set us back along the righteous path! As we puffed our way along mossy switchbacks, as the purple, frail but lovely Rocky Mountain forget-me-nots appeared in finger holds on rocky outcroppings, cairns reassured us. Cairns center us, remind us where we are, guide us gently on our way. As we gained elevation and the adolescent fog lifted, I always marveled at the beautiful significance of cairns along the trails.

On the trail of life, I thank unknown friends for leaving cairns as I suck in breath and take each arduous step toward bagging another peak. How often—in forms I sometimes recognize only later—have I been blessed with signs. People are living cairns on the trails of life. Advice from those who love us—parents, grandparents, trusted friends and elders—act as wayfinders when we stray. In times of great transition and struggle, our connections to one another save us from the abyss and draw us into the glorious gift of life.

As our children hike toward adulthood, may we remember the importance of cairns. May we continue to act as silent guideposts as they journey toward adulthood. Angels on our paths—in the form of family and friends who are there for us when we need them—sanctify our journeys. I am endlessly grateful for my childhood, my family, and the mentors who remind me where my path is when I am lost. Let us be thankful for and let us remember to notice the sacred markers along our way. May we be signals—*signum fidei*, signs of faith—to one another. May the rough stretches of our lives give way to expansive views and better times. And may we all, even with teenagers in the house, even when things seem impossible, remember to take in the scenery and try to enjoy the hike.

Chapter Fifteen

Preschool Teacher
(Rest Them)

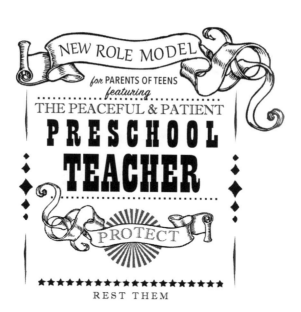

SO TEENAGERS ARE like two-year-olds. Two-year-olds need naps. Sometimes if they're sobbing and breaking down and the world doesn't make sense, insist your adolescent son or daughter take a nap. Offer a teddy bear. Sometimes, even when they're restless, they'll feel grateful and succumb. They'll sleep like rocks and wake up strangely refreshed, full of less despair and more hope. Teenagers need naps, too.

Preschool Teachers make naptime a part of every day. They recognize the early warning signs of tantrums and meltdowns. They also know the cause of wild behavior is often pure exhaustion. They patiently hand out sleeping mats, sweetly read a story or sing a lullaby, whisper "hush" and turn down the lights. Some children slumber and others lie awake, but they are quiet. They rest their bodies, brains and speaking voices. They recharge themselves and gather focus for the remainder of their day. A Preschool Teacher reminds parents how to protect our kids from sensory overload, hyper scheduling and the cacophony of life. The Preschool Teacher knows all important tasks are accomplished best when students are not overtired.

The champion parents I've observed demand some down time for their teenagers. They make a regular habit of rejecting the culture of frantic activity. They find ways to help their families get off the hamster wheel, at least some of the time. Like our new role model the Preschool Teacher, they give their progeny some time to hear their own thoughts, to reflect and recharge.

LET THEM GET BORED.

What an unfamiliar concept boredom can be in this age of constant entertainment and digital distraction! I have an inkling a little tedium during the growing up years may be vital to the development of self-sufficient adults. A Preschool Teacher knows how kids learn to entertain themselves when they must be quiet and when they get a little bored.

They invent games and fanciful stories. They find joyful, surprising things under rocks and seat cushions. They make up songs or find patterns in ceiling tiles or memorize jokes. Too much unstructured boredom, of course, can produce frustration and anger, but a little dose of it now and again forces us all to rely on ourselves and get creative about what to do. Finding ways out of boredom is a fine resource to develop because, let's face it, adulthood so often demands it.

Down time for teenagers, then, should include intervals of solitude and rest. Above all, they should have unplugged time. Neither video games nor bingeing on *The Gilmore Girls* is the kind of respite teenagers need. Nap time is sometimes literally a nap. Sometimes it is free time when nothing is demanded of them and they have few distractions. If we are lucky enough to have access to nature, we can give our teenagers the gift of being alone with themselves among the trees, in the fields or on the shore. The awesome, humbling feeling of insignificance one can feel at the top of a mountain or bottom of a canyon—along with the practice of letting bird calls and leaf shapes fill our days—is tonic to many challenges.

LET THEM PLAY.

The Preschool Teacher knows downtime also looks like recess, another daily part of the preschool gig. Little kids need to play and so do teenagers. Parents can follow this role model when—to protect teenagers from hectic schedules and heavy expectations—we give them time and space to fool around and amuse themselves. We can pay attention to how much our teenagers are playing. I urge you, however, to believe that almost never, at the high school level, does participation in organized sports or music programs give our teenagers the kind of freewheeling downtime we expect from "play." For most teenagers, playing sports (or an instrument) feels much like working a job. I'm a big fan of activities and competition at every level. The benefits are many. But let us not fool ourselves: some of the teenagers most in need of rest, downtime and a chance to play are the kids playing sports (or instruments) with the most vigor and success.

IT'S A FINE LINE.

Once again, we need to step back from every situation and be sure we know what's going on before we can determine what steps (if any) we must take to protect our vulnerable, complicated teenagers. Often, deciding which role model to emulate in the moment requires us to ask the most delicate, perplexing question, "Can I honor my child's unique journey toward adulthood?" Next, the new role models who can help parents of teenagers do exactly that.

ROLE MODELS
WHO HONOR

THE MENTOR
THE ARTIST
THE PEREGRINE FALCON

Chapter Sixteen

Mentor
(Guide Them)

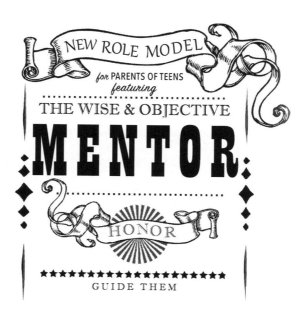

AS WE'VE LEARNED, teenagers are in the midst of actual identity crisis. They are on a heroic quest to define themselves and their roles in the world. Maybe the English Teacher in me loves adolescent people so much because across the ages they are the best protagonists. From Hamlet and David Copperfield to Jane Eyre and Stephen Dedalus, the literary characters who come of age illuminate the adolescent journey. Epic stories of young heroes facing good and evil are as old as time and eternally relevant. Let us turn, then, to the ancient Greeks for parenting inspiration. When Odysseus shipped off for his epic journey, he left the elderly Mentor to care for his son (except it's actually that wily goddess Athena, in yet another disguise). Here is an early example of the Mentor archetype so familiar in the Western canon. When grown-up Telemachus goes in search of his father (to save him from all that globe trotting, monster fighting and nymph imprisonment), Mentor accompanies and guides him. The Mentor character maintains an objective stance, laughs gently at the hero's plight and helps guide younger people to actualization, fullness and adulthood. The Mentor role model instructs parents to breathe deeply, see with non-judgmental eyes, and guide our children to realizing the very best versions of themselves.

We know and love these Mentor characters. They are ubiquitous in Shakespeare, sacred texts and our favorite popular tales. Think of Cinderella's Fairy Godmother, Pinocchio's conscience Jiminy Cricket, Mary Poppins, Yoda, Professor Dumbledore and the mentor-clown of The Lion King, Rafiki. They often talk in riddles. They coax, cajole and tease. We never know their personal agendas; they remain neutral and entertain us as they guide young heroes to self-actualization. Parents, like Mentors, can put our ourselves aside as we try to honor each child's autonomy from our families and independent journey toward adulthood.

PART ONE: LET THEM BE THEMSELVES.

As you may recall, one of the things I hope my children will be able to do before they leave me is establish a unique identity. The reason accomplishing this task is so unpleasant and often painful is because it means—in tangible ways—separating from the family: asserting differences and claiming freedom from Mom and Dad, from the expectations we have of them, even from their own concepts of themselves. They change personalities and loyalties as often as they change their underwear. They reject us and everything we say. And I mean everything.

. . . .

PARENTING CASE STUDY:
Defiance and Difference

I have lately watched one of my favorite 12-year-old girls—precariously close to her first menstrual cycle—go through the changeling-style transformation. Right before her mother and me, she has turned from a dear companion whom we love to take shopping into a surly little thing who rolls her eyes at our advice, our jokes, our fashion choices and our efforts to speak to her at all. Because she is not my own personal child, I am amused by this behavior, so clearly a giant, flashing signal that puberty is upon her. I recognize how perfectly normal she's acting and I never take it personally. Her mother, on the other hand, feels rejected and abused. When she takes a deep breath and remembers how natural and necessary it is for her daughter to do just this—to reject Mom and everything for which she stands—she can laugh a little. We can all laugh a little more when we take a new look at our teenagers and honor their need to be defiant and different from us.

. . . .

Often, the forming of unique identities means our teenagers will choose passions and pursuits different from those we might choose for them. Once again, it gets personal. A child with more talent (academically, musically, athletically, physically) than we had, who is clearly on the path to a stunning college and professional career, may drop the activity in question like a hot potato sometime during the teenage years. It's awfully difficult to remove ourselves—our hopes, dreams, identities and all that money we spent on lessons or equipment—from the equation. It's tough to comprehend why someone's gift or talent does not bring them joy and in fact begins to feel like a terrible burden. Sometimes, though, teenagers wear our ideas about their success or fulfillment like ill-fitting, itchy sweaters. Super precocious kids can be especially challenging in this arena, but even the most typical child may abandon the very thing we are sure will reap great rewards. To honor the unique identity forma-tion of our teenagers, parents need to let them walk their own paths and make their own mistakes, no matter how painful or personal it feels. Remember: the difficulty is not permanent. They do grow up eventually! We look, then, to the Mentor to help us learn how to honor our teen-agers and the unique, individual, challenging process of becoming their very own people. The role models in previous chapters help us know our teenagers. When we've gathered our information, sometimes we must take action to protect them. Other times, though, the next step is to accept what we know so we can honor them enough to guide their way.

If we had to share the physical existence of our teenaged sons and daughters, we couldn't make it through our days. It would involve more sweating, scratching, twitching, and random vocal explosions than adults could stand. When we remember the actual experience of adolescents, it is easier to forgive them for being themselves, for being more fascinated by naughty drawings, farts and insects than homework or hygiene. In the classroom, I was eternally reminded what folly it is to try and push teen-agers beyond the limits of their cognitive or psychosocial development.

Teenagers are hardwired not to care about many of the things their parents find important. They are, in fact—those adolescent brains!—programmed to take risks, challenge rules and act like blithering idiots. I considered myself a great success on many days of teaching adolescents if no one fell out of a chair, broke into fisticuffs or vomited in the classroom. I hated to lower my standards but I had to admit my limits and try to forgive them their human imperfections and adolescent tendencies.

As always, working with teenagers requires the balance of a tightrope walker: don't expect too much but don't sell them short. Honoring teens means holding them responsible for meeting their considerable potential, while at the same time cutting them the slack their physical condition (puberty) demands. Sometimes, a child must sit still and pay attention; other times, the same kid may need a moment of distraction, a lap around the block or the chance to tell a joke out loud. When I found some semblance of balance between my expectations and their pace, my students and I connected. Lightbulbs went off almost visibly above heads. We shared the satisfaction of learning, of *getting it*, if only for a moment. The parents I hold in highest regard find this balance by guiding, forgiving and honoring their teenagers.

To reach adolescents—and to teach them—we do best to honor exactly where they are in the complicated, confusing process of growing up, which sometimes prevents them from meeting our expectations and complicates our relationships with them. When we recognize their age-appropriate behavior and admit their limits, we can guide them and help them feel safer in the uncertain world. Our new role model the Mentor reminds us (once again!) not to get bumped by a teenager's rejection. The Mentor just chuckles and remembers how natural and normal it is. The Mentor has seen it all before and has the distance to find it all a little bit silly.

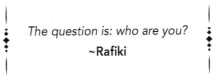

The question is: who are you?
~Rafiki

PART TWO: IT'S NOT YOUR JOB. (LET GO. DELEGATE.)

Developmentally, teenagers seek to differentiate themselves from their parents. They are programmed to reject our advice and rely on the opinions and guidance of others (especially peers). As you may be aware, teenagers value anyone—teachers, coaches, friends, pop stars, neighbors, street preachers, derelicts—more than Dear Old Mom and Dad. Really. Anyone who *isn't their parent* has more cred with our kids than we have. So let us put good mentors in their paths. Know the teachers who influence them; introduce them to music instructors or youth leaders or other adults you trust. If your teenagers show interest in new passions, however haphazard they may seem, do some research. Encourage their fledging interests by introducing them to adults who can guide them (and whom you know to be good people). [3]

. . . .

PARENTING CASE STUDY:
Prom Drama (A Tale of Hurt Feelings)

Angela tried not to weep as her pretty, popular daughter left for Prom. A junior in high school, Bella usually gave her parents no more trouble than one expects from an active teen. A few missed curfews and months of attitude were mitigated by her generally cheerful demeanor and solid work ethic. Bella was excited to be on the Prom court and to arrive on the arm of one of the cutest boys in her class. She and her mom had spent weeks anticipating the big night, sharing pics of the perfect dress, shoes, accessories and hairstyle. Almost nightly Bella kept Angela up too late, gigging and discussing the merits of a French manicure versus a bright pop of color. Angela—aware these moments of concord are all too rare—enjoyed being swept up in the excitement. Bella was a busy girl and her mom didn't mind helping with the Prom preparation. Dress shopping was a joy, a rite of passage, and even the avalanche of details seemed fun. Angela made two trips to the seamstress. She cancelled and rescheduled Bella's nail appointment. She picked up the boutonniere and tied a confetti-filled balloon to a certain car in the school parking lot (why, she was not entirely sure, but her daughter asked and she complied). She solicited every restaurant within five miles for donations to the after-Prom festivities. And then on Prom night itself, Bella casually announced she'd be getting ready at a friend's house. When Angela protested, Bella assured her the friend's mom was better at doing hair and a better photographer than anyone in their family (Angela had to admit, it was true) and would forward all the pictures. She gave her mom a peck on the cheek, promised to be home on time, loaded her finery into the backseat and drove away. Her poor mother stood bewildered on the front porch trying to reconcile her mature years with the distinctly adolescent feeling of being dropped by her best friend.

· ·

If you are lucky, your kids will find Mentors to the do work parents cannot do (because they are not us). Our kids are not biologically compelled to reject every single word their Mentors say. Because they don't have to rebel against these other adults, it's a simpler (and usually more pleasant) relationship. Teachers, coaches and other Mentors see our kids more objectively than we do. Their perspective feels good to a teenager in the midst of a (totally normal, absolutely necessary) identity crisis. Adolescents are more free to try on quirky personae, test off-color jokes or divulge the deepest, shocking secrets of their souls to people who are not their parents. That's just the way it is during these crazy years.

It's easy to feel jealous of these other grown ups. Even when we acknowledge the guidance they give and the value they add to our children's lives, it's tough not to resent them when our kids appear to like them more than they like us. I am begging you: let it go. It's an adolescent's job to need us less and less. If we know and trust the other adults to whom they turn during these years, let us thank our lucky stars! When they call teachers and coaches their "second parents," let us get down on our knees and be grateful for our prodigious fortune; this job is too damned tough to do alone. Parents, please, please make room for all the willing parenting partners who cross your path! Please be strong and sensible enough to share your burden with a willing village.

Of course Angela's feelings of rejection were real—and heartbreaking—but eventually she found solace in her friendship with the other girl's mother, who generously shared the beautiful photos she took of Prom night. Let us be grateful for all the mentors who help us raise our teenagers into responsible adulthood. When we are able, parents do best to act like Mentors, maintaining an objective distance, a healthy sense of humor and a vault full of sound guidance. The truth, however, is that most often adolescents take their cues and their advice from other people. May all our teenagers, as they journey toward meeting the pure potential of their grown-up selves, find Mentors who guide them well and keep them safe from harm.

PARENTING CASE STUDY:
The Trouble with Teachers (in loco parentis)

> **in loco parentis** ˈɪn ˈloʊkoʊ /parentis/
>
> In the place of a parent; allowing institutions such as schools to act in the best interest of a student

Aimee was fit to be tied: her son's violin teacher had lost his patience and his cool before a big competition. Young Christopher (an accomplished musician, up for college scholarships and summer fellowships) had approached the teacher with a complaint—nay, a suggestion! a mere request!—and the teacher had not taken it well. He had, in fact, blown up at Christopher and the kid was devastated. The two have been together for years; the teacher is coach, mentor, therapist, family friend, trusted confidante. He cares as much about Christopher's success as anyone and has guided him brilliantly thus far. But the recent scene at the concert hall had Aimee in knots. As she narrated the ugly confrontation, my educator vision kicked in and I saw the scene from a slightly different perspective: the teacher's.

I'm sharing here what I said to Aimee because she appreciated the new point of view. Maybe it will help you, too. As you know, I recommend forgiving our children for being adolescents and acting their age. I also insist we parents forgive ourselves. And now I shall remind you how important it is to forgive the villagers helping to raise our children. Even when there is no jealousy—when the parents of a teenager love and trust the Mentor—the relationship can be complicated, challenging and demanding of sprawling forgiveness. Christopher's violin teacher temporarily lost his distance, his objective stance. Christopher's request in fact was a signal of his burgeoning independence. He needs less instruction from his coach at competitions these days (because he has been prepared so well for so many years). His teacher reacted much like a parent would. He felt threatened and insulted by his student not needing him. He felt challenged. The teacher had in fact become in loco parentis when it came to the violin. When I pointed this out to Aimee, I watched relief sweep over her face and body. The teacher had almost immediately been contrite and embarrassed by his reaction, so healing had already begun for all of them, but looking at it from the teacher's point of view helped everything make more sense for my friend and her gifted son.

Throughout every school year, I urge parents to remember teachers are people too (as are coaches, club leaders, grandparents, trainers . . .). When they are especially invested in our children's lives, it gets personal. When one of these blessed Mentors acts badly, let us first consider things from their side of the street. And then, always—of course—let us investigate further and know what's going on. We have no tolerance for abuse, emotional torture or dangerous behavior by adults in positions of trust. But it's worth considering and honoring the relationships longtime Mentors build with our offspring. If they are truly invested in our kids, they are probably emotionally and personally entangled on some level (much like parents). We should demand positive, healthy, life-affirming relationships. Absolutely. But if every now and again "good" teachers or coaches seem to go off the deep end, let's consider the possibility that our goofy, complicated kids might have pushed them. And, within reason and the bonds of human decency, let's try to forgive them.

Remember, teachers and coaches are vital resources. They help us know our kids. If a student struggles in class, a vigilant teacher (and most of them are; trust me; they wouldn't do their thankless jobs if they didn't love those kids) will let you know. A teacher will present the actual struggle, which may differ from anything we have previously known about our child. No adult I have ever met relishes a confrontation about cheating, plagiarism, laziness, or bullying. It costs a teacher to call a student onto the carpet or to call parents with unsettling news. Parents who respond with "not my baby" and "she's just not challenged in your class" miss a vital opportunity. Teenagers try on new personae and labels as frantically as they change their outfits before the mirror on Saturday night. The people they are at school may not resemble the people who come home to us. If we remember to open our ears and hearts and honor the teacher-student relationship, Mentors will help us honor our children and their process of growing up.

. . . .

Five Ways to Thank Your Child's Mentors

Remember chipping in for—even hand-crafting—gifts for your child's elementary school teachers, back when everybody liked kids and everything was more precious in every way? In most upper grades across America, this lovely habit is abandoned. I understand why: all those teachers, all that parental exhaustion, all the over-scheduled hyped-up craziness of our lives! Gestures of appreciation for middle and high school teachers are never expected but always appreciated. It's thankless work, y'all. Here are a few quick ways to make a difference in the lives of beleaguered secondary school teachers and others who spend time with our teens:

1. Invest in several $5 or $10 gift cards from local coffee shops or bakeries. I know parents who keep a stash in the glove compartment, ready to toss appreciatively to a teacher on a rough day or a coach who has stayed late to work with their kid.

2. Express your gratitude, formally, to their supervisors. A letter to the principal or school board about a particularly great teacher

159

will make a lovely addition to a personnel file. If coaches or instructors run their own small businesses, send an email full of evidence and soundbites about how much they've helped your kid. Invite them to quote you for promotional purposes.

3. Remind your kids to say "thank you." Several students in my teaching career practiced the lovely habit of regularly calling, "Thank you!" over their shoulders as they left my classroom. I remember every single one of these kids with great affection. What a difference it made to me, after struggling through another lesson on another endless day!

4. Check back. When your child does something—even months or years later—that would make that teacher, coach or other mentor especially proud, share the news. Let the adults know what a difference they made. My husband recently received a call from a boy he'd coached from the ages of eight to 12. Now a senior in high school, the young man just signed to play baseball with a good college and he called to thank one of his first coaches for getting him there. Classy move. Mentors feel not only proud but vindicated when they hear about their students wising up, making sound choices and accomplishing great things.

5. Ask your teenagers to write notes of thanks. No matter how brief or awkward, no matter mistakes in spelling or punctuation, these notes are kept and cherished forever. I happen to know.

PROFESSIONAL HELP: WHEN AND HOW SHOULD WE GET IT?

Once in a while, a teenager gets truly lost and needs support beyond what parents and the immediate community can give. They may require a more formal, professional kind of Mentor to help them find their way. Parents who know what's going on and who have determined something must be done to protect a teen from real and present danger may realize a need for professional help to honor their child's journey. Two questions surface in this case: how do we determine when it's time for professional help and how do we go about getting it? Our new role models and our conviction to stay vigilant help us find some balance as we walk this tightrope. Sometimes we lean into our teenagers' strife; other times we step back and let them make their own mistakes.

It is not always possible, by the way, to force human beings to get help even when they desperately need it. But we can make sure to get help for ourselves. I'm a fan of Woody Allen movies and therefore regular psychotherapy, for myself and as many members of my family who will cooperate. Even in easy times, I tell them, life is hard. The crazy people are the ones who think they can do it alone, without an analyst. With various measures of buy-in, my own kids have accepted my attempts to normalize this form of mentorship. They don't go constantly, but they do say things like, "Mom, I'm feeling sad and I don't know why. Can I go see the therapist?" It comforts me to know they have a professional Mentor, a sounding board, a place to go and express their darkest fears. When they suffer trauma—either profound or mundane—they are already in conversation with a professional they trust to help them make sense of things and begin to heal. If you or your family are less enthusiastic about spilling your guts to strangers, I remind you once again how important your village is. Coaches, teachers, family, friends and clerks at the local market can give support to your kids and important information to you when your teenagers are in trouble. The best of Mentors—theirs and

161

ours—maintain a healthy distance, let kids express their goofy selves but sound the alarm when they see signs of real danger.

If your family won't go to therapy but you think it might help you, go alone. If your health suffers because you need help relaxing, gaining perspective and forgiving yourself, get that help. Take yoga, Pilates, or meditation classes. Do a craft if it comforts you. Go to church or a support group or an acupuncturist. Please try to do whatever you need to do to stay healthy because raising teenagers takes every bit of your strength (more on this concept in the third section of the book). Meanwhile, back to those kids. . . .

When we wonder if a child needs professional help, parents can ask those familiar, fundamental questions. Do we know what's going on? If a teenager gets into trouble—with school, the law, substance abuse, other people—it is more important than ever to gather the facts as best we can and see the problem clearly. Must we protect our child from real and present danger? If we've determined the need for action, what does it look like? We might try many approaches, inspired by each of our new role models, before we find the best solution. Can we honor our teenager's unique identity formation? Can we forgive their faults and foibles, check our own pride and put our kids in the right hands?

Professional intervention is necessary in some cases, generally understood as when a child is in danger of doing harm to self or others. Let's walk through the process of stepping back and asking:

1. Do we know what's going on with our kids? Our new role models the Falcon, Private Investigator and Ninja inspire us to get to the bottom of things and accept the bitter truth of the situation. If we learn about adolescents with serious substance-abuse problems, who cut, starve or otherwise mutilate themselves, who hurt animals or other human

beings, who feel suicidal or who break serious laws, we must take swift and decisive action to keep them safe.

2. Must I protect my teenager from real and present danger? In these extreme cases, professional intervention may be the logical solution: treatment or rehabilitation, the care of medical doctors, community service, even boarding school. When a kid needs to be rescued from harm, we turn to our new role models the Soldier and the Personal Trainer for guidance. In less acute cases, when the danger is not so imminent, when they need shelter, strong arms, rest and play, we may look to the Tree or our two teachers—English and Preschool—to know what to do. We can't always force kids to get help but we can leave a trail of breadcrumbs to help them to find their own way.

3. Can I honor my child's unique journey? Saving teens from trouble and helping them heal is, like all of parenting, messy and imperfect. If parents know we've stepped in as much as feels appropriate and secured professional help for ourselves and our children, let's try to trust the process, make changes, forgive, forget, and move forward.

When adolescents are in acute need of professional help, it is fairly easy for parents to find resources. Schools, community centers and private companies offer ready help and the comfort of knowing you're not alone. If you feel truly in the dark, search the internet or reach out to a trusted member of your tribe just to get the ball rolling. Although they're not always pleasant, there are ready options available for these teens and their families. I am sorry to say that when a child's battles are less critical, the options for help are less obvious and more difficult to find. Oh, my friends, it can be a lonely road, walking through the wilderness with a struggling adolescent! It can touch so many personal wounds and fears! Parents feel as lost as their kids! Again I remind you how important it is to seek balance. Look to our new role models and take healthy approaches to the problem. Keep juggling; keep seeking; try and try again. If one course of action falls short of helping your teenager, try another. Trust your gut when advice from other adults knocks you off the tightrope. Get back on; lean in a different direction without upsetting your own balance; stay flexible. It's a wobbly, precarious, often scary equilibrium but our kids are worth it. Above all—in this chapter about Mentors—I hope you won't go through it completely alone. I hope you will reach out, professionally or person-ally, to someone besides all the voices in your head. I hope you will find a counselor-confessor who will nod and comfort you and let you know you've got everything it takes to do this job.

Should you fret about burdening your community when you ask for help, fear not. I guarantee you'll have plenty of opportunity to pay it forward. Someday soon—really!—you will be out of this thicket and able to laugh. You'll gain a wise perspective. You'll recognize the familiar, frustrating patterns of adolescence and you'll cast light into the darkness for younger, more hapless parents. Ah, the circle of life!

Our job, guided by our new role model the Mentor, is to honor our children and lead them to themselves. This means recognizing the things they love and are good at, which make them feel happy and fulfilled, which might be different than the things we think they are good at or want them to do. Even when we acknowledge the many benefits of parenting like a Mentor, it's difficult work requiring awesome forgiveness. We turn, then, to our next new role model, who reminds us how to forgive.

Chapter Seventeen

Artist
(Forgive Them)

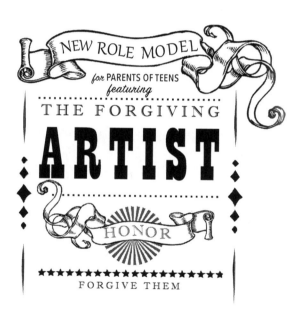

IF YOU HAVE ever been involved in a creative process you may have said, "close enough for jazz" or its visual companion, "call it art." These are phrases uttered by creative people who have put their souls into something, who know their creation is far from perfect but who also believe the wisdom of calling it imperfect but good enough. Indeed, when we think of a jazz musician or an Artist, we might picture someone with patience who understands the messiness of the process, who treats mistakes with a sense of humor, who has the creativity to see flaws and find beauty in them. Our new role model the Artist instructs us to expect the process of growing up to be messy, imperfect and slightly amusing.

. . . .

Kintsugi: There Is a Crack in Everything

In Japan, traditional ceramic artists employ a technique called *kintsugi.* They restore broken bowls by filling the cracks with gold. The rich symbolism is intentional; they believe the history and scars of a vessel make it more valuable. *Kintsugi* is a meditation on imperfection, inviting us to believe our weaknesses and broken-ness are indeed our most beautiful parts. What an important message to convey to our teenagers, who feel so broken in so many confusing ways!

. . . .

Despite all we have discussed and all signs to the contrary, our expectations and opinions matter to our teenagers. We would never know it based on much of their behavior but they deeply long to please us and make us proud. Certain wise people believe expectations are disappointments waiting to happen. Parental expectations, along with the glossy perfection of the media, can make teenagers feel diminished and inadequate. Remember, they are hormonally compelled to *not* be perfect. They are set up for failure—for disappointing us and falling short of expectations—every time they turn around. Our new role model the Artist reminds us to honor our adolescents by letting them know we expect them to stumble and fall because it's a natural part of life, and by helping them finds creative ways to deal with failure and struggle.

DON'T TELL THEM WHO THEY ARE.

Over and over, I see my own children and my students—well into their twenties, I am sorry to report—reject the expectations and labels their parents give them. They even (sometimes especially) rebel against the positive monikers we ascribe, thinking we are bolstering their self-esteem. The "bright kid," the "brilliant musician," the "prodigy," also the "honest" or "responsible" child will, upon hitting puberty, cultivate some identity directly opposed to the one his parents have created for him. Nobody manifests the conundrum more publicly than "professional" children (say, Miley Cyrus or Lindsay Lohan). More than I care to remember, I have seen students blow huge opportunities, sabotage scholarship offers or throw Advanced Placement tests in erroneous attempts to assert their independence to people they think control their lives.

We should try not to tell our kids who we think they are. They don't want to hear it. Think of how often we inadvertently tell them what they think, and how our words sound to them. Our kids name a "mean" classmate and we respond, "Oh, you've known her since you were three! She's not mean, she's just irritating you!" They hear, "Your opinions and feelings are wrong." We state facts about their lives, "My daughter is competing in State this weekend." They hear us bragging, glorifying a catalog of irrelevant achievements that cannot possibly define them. We gently make a request, "Could you please remember to close the pantry door?" They hear, "Why can't you do anything right?" We have to walk on eggshells and maintain that elusive balance when attempting to reach the human beings wrapped inside our adolescent children. They are hyper sensitive.

No doubt about it. It's best not to define them at all. We should listen, however, when they define themselves.

LISTEN WHEN THEY TELL US WHO THEY ARE.

When adolescents divulge their secrets, I am stunned by their simultaneous longing for parents who really know them and their compulsion to develop covert personalities. They resent us for not understanding them yet they make it impossible to understand them. It's exhausting. Teenagers speak in weird codes, at midnight when we are heading at last for bed, through idiotic fashion choices and late assignments and their terrible choices in friends. They speak to us when they throw temper tantrums and lose their minds over relationships and lie about their whereabouts and shoot airsoft guns into windows. Whatever cryptic messages they send, we do best to curb our desires to label them.

Let them speak to us, define themselves to us. Try not to be afraid. Trust your children; you've raised them well. They have freedom within boundaries and all the skills they need to navigate the rough waters of growing up. Nothing they do could ever really shame you; let them know they are okay in your eyes, no matter what. The whole wide world judges and mocks and challenges a teenager; let *us* be a safe place where they can express every little impulse they have without fear of being cut out of the will. Try not to mock them when they do predictable things. Try not to visibly roll your eyes (it's hard!). Try to listen more than tell.

When our teenagers tell us who they are and who they want to be, we can watch them flourish. We can see them blossom in ways that will profoundly surprise us. Let us honor each child's journey to happy, responsible adulthood: each personal, different from ours, unexpected, singular, beautiful journey. When our teenagers are in real and present danger, let us know it and swoop in to save them. Let us give them freedom within boundaries which protect them. Let us honor their own mystifying, complicated expressions of the people they long to be.

BUT NOT WHEN THEY DESCRIBE US.

It's important to let teenagers describe themselves and define their roles in the world but it is madness to let them describe or define us. Teenagers (due to no fault of their own) cannot be trusted to know their own minds; they are unsure and indecisive but full of passionate conviction. They equivocate, waver, vacillate and throw ridiculous tantrums. Never, never let them draw you into their insanity. And no matter what you do, don't trust anything they say about you. They might accuse you of being an overzealous supporter one day and an absent, abusive parent the next. Teenagers will say anything, to anybody, when they're frustrated or lost or caught in a power struggle.

Let's all make ourselves a deal. Let's not listen to a thing our children utter about us until they are about three months into their first year of parenting their own kid. If we honor their innate process of differenti-ating, defining and destroying, we'll see a different version of ourselves through their grown-up eyes. In the eyes of the adult, responsible people we hope each of our children becomes, we're gonna look just fine. We've got a long journey ahead. If we start practicing detachment now, adoles-cent insults will slide right off.

FORGIVE OURSELVES.

Our first child's dramatic entrance into the world set the tone of total disorientation. Rushing down the hospital hallway toward emergency surgery, I wailed to my husband, "But I didn't read the chapters about c-sections!" Nothing about parenting is what we expect. We diligently prepare for every challenge we can imagine, only to meet trials we have not fathomed. A couple I know are raising their *fifth* teenager. The older four are happy, healthy, well-adjusted adults who make their parents proud. And yet my friend, like so many of us, is at her wits' end. She recently confessed, "It's like we've never done this before!" It seems the current teenager is busy devising brand new ways to rebel, challenge authority, express his youthful angst. These parents are seasoned professionals. They thought they knew every trick in the book. But every day with every teenager reminds us there *is* no book. No rules, no rhyme or reason . . . it really is like a carnival funhouse: the familiar gets distorted into a terrifying new reality.

Every time I consult a parent of older children, I am comforted. Their wisdom—and their distance from the desperate insanity of living with adolescents—gives me hope. They say things like, "Oh, please," and "That's nothin'" and they laugh out loud at my petty concerns.

. . . .
PARENTING CASE STUDY:
This is the First Time I've Done This!

One of the fine people offering me comfort is Karen Dawson Haag, mother of real-life grown ups (and former teenagers). She offered this parenting gem in response to one of my blog posts. I am honored she's allowed me to share it here.

"I had an a-ha moment when raising my oldest. One day, my teenager and I were having an argument about who-knows-what. I suddenly said, 'Hey! This is the first time I've raised a child and you have to cut me some slack.'

That broke the mood and we laughed. Sometimes, just telling your kids that you have fears, you don't know what you're doing, you love them and think you're looking out for them, and you're open to hearing their ideas made all the difference for us. Now, we both say, Hey! This is the first time I've done this. Help me." [4]

Here is some real wisdom. What a gift Karen gave her teenagers when she admitted she didn't know what she was doing! When parents admit we are struggling, when we reveal our weaknesses, when we ask for forgiveness, we invite our children into the truth. As always, it's a balance: we need to remain strong and assure them we will protect them, but we gain their trust when we also tell them we don't quite know how. We should strive not to burden our kids with our own struggles but to remain transparent when we're thrown off balance.

Karen also underscores the value of laughing at ourselves. Sometimes (often) with teenagers, laughter is all we've got. "Breaking the mood" is magic. If we forget to laugh, we succumb to anger and frustration. If we can find the comedy in the situation, it's easier to forgive ourselves and our children and the whole, wide world. It is also true that as our kids get older, it's harder to laugh at them and at ourselves. I beg you to try because laughter is one of the languages we can speak with teens. The conundrum is how unfunny it gets and how unenjoyable they can be once puberty hits.

Life is a tragedy in close-up but a comedy in long-shot. To truly laugh, you must be able to take your pain and play with it.
~Charlie Chaplin

FORGIVE OUR PARENTS.

Now is probably a good time to pause and try to feel benevolent toward the people who raised us. A bit of forgiveness for the mom who took such a militant stance against video games her son couldn't control his habit once he left the house. A nod of sympathy to the father who wanted so strongly to protect his daughter from worrying about money he neglected to teach her responsible spending habits. Sure, our parents were imperfect and they messed us up. But if we look through the lens of mercy, it's often easy to believe (even if it is only way, deep down) their intentions were good. During the raging storm of adolescence, it behooves us to take this pause and remember—no matter how it seemed, no matter how awful they were—parents generally do the best they can. Sometimes as their children we think, "Well, their best wasn't good enough," but lifelong resentments make our own parenting more difficult. We may set out to do better than our parents did; often, we overcorrect and send the cosmic pendulum swinging in precisely the opposite direction. As we pause for this moment of forgiveness and understanding, let us also consider the effect our rebellion and resentment might have had on the people who raised us.

OUR PARENTS PROBABLY MEANT WELL.

I think about the parents who place a great premium on their daughter's modesty. Sure, it feels repressive, prude and provincial to the child, but her costume of defiance (booty shorts and bondage sandals) represents something more pernicious than teenaged sass to her Mom and Dad. I recall the stoic father who shed tears as his 19-year-old son hitchhiked away from the family farm, off for adventure and parts unknown (in the days before cell phones and easy communication). Listen. I was the truculent teenager in these stories every time—the female Prodigal Son, pugnacious by nature—hellbent on breaking every boundary my parents set for me. I take the side of the riotous adolescent more often than I should at my age. But when I see it now from the parents' point of view it breaks my heart. What feels like oppression to a teenager is often a parent's purest form of love. We want to keep our kids safe—their spirits, their souls, their lives—because we love them more deeply than we knew it was possible to love. Hey, I'm not your therapist, and how much forgiveness you extend to your parents at this stage of the game is up to you. I'm just saying it's probably worth it to consider the spirit (rather than the specifics) of their purpose when they raised us.

FORGIVENESS IS A SACRED ACT.

One typical arena of teenaged mutiny is the church or temple. Developmentally, our children's rebellion and insolence is appropriate and expected. It's all part of their weird, wonderful process of establishing autonomy. Adolescent impulsivity and sensitivity—especially to pleasure and rewards—are in overdrive. Religious services and doctrines, meanwhile, are boring, predictable and stifling. Teenagers think and feel deeply but their brains are all over the place. They become amateur (and annoying) philosophers. By definition, teenagers don't like being told what to do or think. Anything from organized religion to family yoga class can feel to teenagers like thought police. Their kneejerk response is to question, then reject, every word adults speak to them. It's normal, then, to spurn the formal structures in which their parents have (consciously and lovingly, I might add) raised them. We do expect it. Intellectually, we even encourage it: no faith is worth much without healthy skepticism. On the other hand, a child's rejection of the saints and angels can send devoted parents into a tailspin of fear and worry. Despite what teenagers think, the parents who haul them to services and *shul* are rarely intent on mind control. We hope instead to give our kids a good foundation, structure in the chaos, a sense of community and a decent set of rules by which to live. Quite likely parents are also concerned with some version of consciousness, or the life force of the child, whatever the source and shape of their faith. We care about our children, whatever we believe about right, wrong or the afterlife. When teenagers turn away, parents worry about their souls, their character and their ability to be good human beings. A teenager's rejection, mockery or profanity can take a deeply personal toll on a parent's psyche. Our new role model the Artist helps us tap the source of forgiveness and honor each child's difficult, rocky road toward her own understanding of the Divine. When they reject our values, they're hoping for a reaction. They want to shock us and maybe even scare us. The best course is to sail on, unmoved by their attempts to rock the boat. Forgive them their attitudes and trust they'll mature in good time. If it helps you, pray for them. A lot.

> Ring the bells that still can ring
> Forget your perfect offering
> There is a crack in everything
> It's how the light gets in.
>
> **~Leonard Cohen**

Chapter Eighteen

Peregrine Falcon
(Push Them)

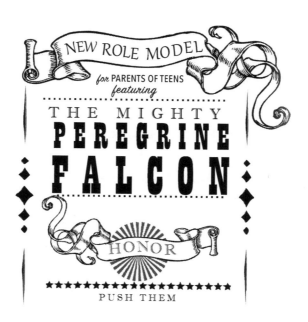

EVERY ONCE IN a while (happily, more often than not), I hear from a student who struggled in high school, who has found a way to light a candle and forgo all the cursing of the darkness. Maybe we have coffee or a meal, and I see a new person before me: mature, responsible, living in the truth and giddy with all the promise the world holds. The child I worried about, prayed for, fought with, cursed and cared for has spun dross into gold more beautiful than I could have conceived. Another amazing thing has happened over the years. Exactly one-third of the students who failed my senior English class—which prevented them from graduating on time—have returned to thank me. One-third of the people who hated, blamed and pleaded with me have returned to say, "It was the best thing you could have done for me." In my mind, I dump the big tub of Gatorade on my own head and do a dance that would get me kicked out of the end zone. And so it goes: they do grow up. They do come around. Their clarity reinforces two inherent qualities of teenagers: they (along with all human beings of any age) seek boundaries and nothing short of real consequences for our actions will help us learn real lessons.

It all comes right back to our role model the Mother Falcon. It's her job to force her children to be independent when the time comes. She regurgitates food and places it down their hungry little necks when they are helpless infants, but as soon as they are old enough to hunt on their own, it gets real. Never mind what she does when it's time to fly: she shoves those babies right out of the nest and watches them fall, struggle and freak out until they spread their own wings and soar. Require your kids to face consequences. Real ones. Like, if you don't flap your wings you will fall to your death.

PARENTING CASE STUDY:
The Beautiful Agony of Consequences

A young man in Denver, Colorado rushed home one afternoon to put the final touches on a scholarship application, due that very day at 4:00 PM. This high school junior is mature, well-spoken, bright. He does well in school, plays sports, works a steady job. He knows a lot of things about the world, but he didn't know (until this particular afternoon) about the importance of time zones.

This intrepid boy submitted his online application at 2:08 PM, happily in advance of his 4:00 deadline. His email was immediately rejected; the application process was closed; the website went blank. The deadline, of course, was 4:00 PM Eastern Standard Time (whereas our unwitting hero lives in the Mountain Time Zone). He missed out on the promise of a dream by eight minutes.

His mama might have lectured or blown her top. You can bet she envisioned thousands of dollars circling right down the drain; I am certain she has repeated, "eight lousy minutes" in varying tones of dismay to all her friends. Instead, she recognized the shock and disappointment in her baby's eyes. She saw the resignation and regret—familiar to cynical adults—which fester when doors slam shut. She knew no one was sorrier than her son about the opportunity he had just missed. Instead of chiding him, instead of frantically emailing powerful people to finagle an extension, she took a deep breath along with him and carried on.

The lessons he learned were many, in that moment and in the following days. Natural consequences are a bitch. He will prob-ably be more careful about deadlines—and time zones—hereafter. He is practicing the art of handling disappointment. Because he is young and gifted and because the world is bountiful, he will have countless other opportunities. He faced frustration, panic and anger at himself and survived. He learned these feelings—like all feelings—are temporary. To my way of thinking, this is a valuable lesson for adolescents to learn. Feelings are temporary.

LIFE LESSONS COST EVEN MORE THAN PIANO LESSONS. PAY HAPPILY.

Wise parents of little kids try to *enjoy* watching their children make stupid mistakes. They know the natural consequences of these actions will produce exactly the results parents desire. Kids will remember their coats if they have felt the chill of forgetting them, or their lunches if they have felt hunger pangs at noon. When the stakes are lower, we can force ourselves to giggle and think, "what a great learning opportunity!" Parents of teenagers, let's try to do the same. Let's try to enjoy watching teenagers face the music, be responsible, suffer the consequences of their idiotic actions. Nothing less will save them from themselves.

When parents rush to solve their problems and rescue them from natural consequences, we deny our children the gift of learning how to fail. It is agonizing, watching our kids suffer the results of their actions, but it is worth it. Every single time, they grow and learn and take one giant leap toward responsible adulthood. As it is with toddlers, some natural consequences make the whole family suffer but we know we have to follow through with the punishment we've promised. When the kindergartener does not, in fact, eat the eight-dollar mac and cheese she ordered—despite threats of no meals out for a whole month—the family eats in for 30 days. When teenagers push their boundaries or fail to hold up their end of certain bargains, they might miss out on opportunities for which parents have already paid. Ouch. Whether it's a dance, concert, or exotic trip denied, it can be an expensive lesson. It can be tempting for parents to go back on their threats and renegotiate gentler (cheaper) sentences. As much as we can, parents, stay strong. If it hurts us, it probably hurts them even more. Consider it an investment in their future. We pay happily for piano lessons; pay cheerfully for life lessons, too.

PARENTING CASE STUDY:
What Teenagers Can Learn When They Get Lost

Kids who drive are a daily lesson in letting go. Since my boys became licensed drivers, I run a constant montage of the Buddha, the Blessed Mother, and Joan Baez in my head while I try to remember to breathe. Thus, when our two teenagers left on a gorgeous November morning for a hike with the wrestling team, it did not occur to me to miss them until well after nightfall. They have a built-in buddy system. They play the same sports and share friends, schedules and a car. Between them, there are two cell phones with healthy data plans, so we trust we'll hear from one when the other is in crisis. Then both their phones went dead. It got cold. My husband remembered telling them to take jackets as they breezed out the door that morning, in shorts and hoodies, calling, "We're fine!"

No parent wants to hear the words "Search and Rescue" but we did. The scanners caught it; the local news ran it: "Wrestling Team Lost in National Forest. No Known Injuries." We were told to report to the Incident Command Post, an hour away over a dark mountain pass. The kids were fine. We knew they were fine. Our hearts quickened, to be sure, but we never truly panicked. It was, however, a stunning reminder . . . of a whole lot of things. Here are some actual lessons our children learned that day. When teenagers get lost—physically or metaphorically—they stand to learn similar, important lessons about life itself.

1. **Anything Can Happen.** Our children have hunter safety licenses, winter-preparedness training and compact emergency kits of their very own. They also possess hats with built-in flashlights, failsafe fire starters and enough warm gear to outfit a dogsled team. None of which they took with them on their warm, November hike. Perhaps they learned a little bit about how important it is to be prepared, because it's impossible to know what might happen.

2. **It is Easy to Lose the Trail.** That's all they did. They were never more than a couple of miles from a road, but their three-hour tour (like Gilligan's) began to seem endless. The trail signs told them they were hiking miles and miles in the wrong direction. Darkness. Forest. They got lost. Like teenagers so often do.

3. **Sometimes, It's Best to Call for Help.** Their coach—a young man whom we trust and respect—called 911 at a clearing with cellular access. On his own or with a buddy, he would have soldiered on and eventually made his way back to the trailhead. But with 11 teenagers in his charge, he made a prudent decision. They stayed put; they called for help. They lit a fire and stayed warm. Coach had extra sandwiches and a few extra pairs of gloves in his pack. He gave them a fine, adult example of being humble and sensible enough to ask for help when we need it.

4. **Good People Will Rescue You.** It's hard for this girl, brought up in the Catholic church, not to pause at the three good souls who came with flashlights, jackets and hot apple cider to rescue the team. A Trinity of volunteers—who left their own family gatherings to venture out into the cold—led the team through the brush, bushwhacking and shouting encouragement, to a

waiting cadre of rescue vehicles and eventually to their happy parents.

5. **Near Falls and Close Calls: We Get to Learn from Our Mistakes.** In wrestling, an almost pin earns "near fall" points which might eventually win the match. The bottom wrestler, on the other hand, gets a second chance to escape the finality of a pin and adjust strategy mid-match. If he learns well, he has a chance to best his opponent. My boys once accused me of "loving it when teenagers get in trouble." In a way, it's true. I love moments like *this*—getting lost in the woods, enough to be frightened, but not injured. The police interrupting a high school party before anyone over imbibes. A 'D' in middle school math which wakes a kid up to how much she really *does* care about her grades. Near falls. Almost pins. Chances to learn, adjust and recover from mistakes before they cause real, life-altering damage.

Every experience is a chance to help young people learn, to guide them, to have family discussions, forge new relationships, test personal limits, and make changes which (we hope) will prevent future missteps.

. . . .

And so, while they are strong but vulnerable, not grown but almost, let us thank Mama Bear for how she has served us but let us leave her to her hibernation, look to our new role models and re-engage. Let us love our teenagers enough to help them become the adults we want them to be. It is worth it.

When our adolescent children start to round the corner back toward the light (and toward us), well, Dear Friends, there is no sweeter feeling in the world.

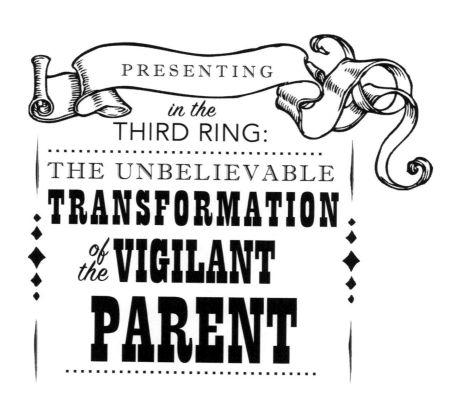

PRESENTING

in the
THIRD RING:

THE UNBELIEVABLE

TRANSFORMATION

of the VIGILANT

PARENT

Chapter Nineteen

The Rewards of Vigilant Parenting: What's in It for You

If we do not transform our pain,
we will most assuredly transmit it.
~Richard Rohr

WE'VE LOOKED AT what's going on with our teenagers; now let's take a look at what's going on with us. While we are learning to know, protect and honor our children, let's do the same for ourselves. When we're engaged in hot conflict with our kids, it's worth taking a candid look at our feelings and reactions: if I know what's going on, I may have to admit that my child reminds me in some way of myself or something unpleasant about my own upbringing and I may be responding from an emotional place. Can I protect my child from my own issues, fears, wounds and anger? Which means I will try to honor my kid enough to step back, recognize the patterns of family life and adolescence and try not to overreact. Parenting with open eyes, strong arms and full hearts helps this nearly impossible job of ours make a little more sense. I hope to convince you in this section what's in it for you.

1. HAPPY RETIREMENT

My husband and I love our kids but we hope to spend our retirement golfing and basking in the sun, not parenting eternal adolescents. Don't misunderstand me: we will always be there for them. We just hope they're able to take care of *us* eventually. Unless we recommit to our children and agree to raise them with the same vigilance and care that marked the toddler years, they might not grow into responsible adults. Experts for generations agree that when the tasks of adolescence are interrupted, children struggle to meet their full potential and complete the process of growing up. We tend to repeat mistakes and patterns of reckless behavior well into adulthood when we don't resolve them during adolescence (Steinberg, 2014). My observations (and my own peculiar life) have convinced me it's true. If parents don't try to find balance on the high wire of raising our families, teenagers might never learn to handle responsibility or make decisions that are healthy for them. Do you know what this means for us? If we throw our hands up (or hibernate) during the adolescent era, our kids might never grow up. Do you see where I'm going with this? Let me put it gracefully: if we stay alert for their few remaining years under our roof, we reduce the likelihood of our children living in our basements when they are 35 years old. It's a solid investment.

As my husband and I lurch toward that empty nest, when our days are shaped by more of our own desires and less by our children's schedules, we can see the light at the end of this godawful tunnel. Strengthened by stories of teens who transform from awkward, misguided kids into adults who do well and do good in the world, we live in hope. Blessed by witnessing our own teenagers' gradual reappearance in the land of the living, we're starting to trust our efforts have been worthwhile. (Parenting almost adults during the college years is, we are learning, a fresh new hell, but the subject of a whole other book!) It is a joyful thing indeed to see children begin to make some sense of their purpose. I don't believe our job is ever done, but as adolescence lifts and our beloved children reappear, the rewards are richer than we imagined (even back when they still smelled nice and wore superhero costumes).

2. A SECOND CHANCE

Teenagers who remind me of myself at their age are always the most difficult for me. I can see their struggles with laser clarity. I recognize their patterns. Often, I understand their behavior but I can't figure out how to help them when they need it. When I am able to remove my *self* from the equation, to step back and guide them with the detachment of a Mentor and the forgiveness of an Artist—which often means admitting my own weaknesses and finding other people who do know how to help them—I get to see young people grow. I get to see them face and overcome challenges I am still working on in my late forties. I'm telling you, this is the greatest secret and greatest reward of parenting: if we let them, teenagers will help us heal our own wounds. We will understand and accept ourselves more fully when the people who remind us of ourselves grow into responsible adults capable of making good decisions. When we can transform our own adolescent angst, recognize it as ours and work diligently to stay out of our children's way, parenting adolescents into adulthood can be the most redeeming thing we've ever done. For our kids and for us, it is worth it to stay awake.

I'm asking you to do a lot, staying vigilant during the roughest years. I hope I have convinced you it's worth it. Here are some thoughts on how to do it and come out on the other side with not only a healthier child but a better, healthier version of yourself, as well.

187

Chapter Twenty

(Know Yourself)
Pitfalls, Roadblocks and the
Circle of Life

AS YOU ARE no doubt aware by now, I believe in frequent Keepin'-It-Real checks for parents of teenagers. As often as I remind you to know the specifics of your children's existence, I'm going to beg you to consider the big picture, too. There are some pretty enormous forces at work in the family circus and in our own lives. Many of them are way beyond our control but if we know what's going on we have a better shot at finding our balance. To that end, let's take a look at the pendulum of parenting.

We are pretty adept at recognizing the child who drives us especially crazy because "she's just like me." We may also readily understand the opposite, a child so unlike us we feel bewildered. We may not so easily recognize other dynamics, including how much our kids may start to remind us of our own parents. It's a thing, folks. Believe it or not, one of the first major disruptions to family harmony often comes in the form of a kid who appears to turn out—or to treat us—"just like my mother!" When children unknowingly act in some way like their grandparents, it can drive us crazy in a terribly specific way. The eldest son takes his ever-loving time to tell a story (just like Grandpa) or the middle daughter is agonizingly sensitive to teasing (just like Grandma). It's a regular old mindbender when our teenagers remind us of the parents who annoyed us when we were teenagers ourselves.

Again with the funhouse mirrors. It's like a layer of irony wrapped in a conundrum of identity formation. We first swing the parent pendulum when we vow never to do as our parents did. Generation to generation, we produce a legacy of opposites. Rigid families produce free love hippies, whose children turn into gun-toting conservatives, who in turn breed the next crop of bleeding-heart do-gooders. If your son or daughter has ever reminded you more of your father or mother than your younger self, take heart. You're not alone. It's all perfectly normal (and really, when you think about it, symmetrical: the universal call and response of becoming human). Our instincts to correct our parents' mistakes—to swing the pendulum—is also natural. It's good. It's evidence of hope, of agency, of believing how we raise our children matters. And it does. Our actions and belief systems shape our children even when the shape they take is exactly opposite of what we envisioned.

My own family of origin moved around a lot while I was growing up. My parents didn't consciously choose a nomadic lifestyle but I got used to being the new kid at school every couple of years. It was hard, renegotiating playground society in every new town, but I thought it made me tough, resilient, adaptable. Still, I mourned the permanent hearth and the friends since kindergarten I never had. I have felt pretty good about letting roots grow for my children. Unlike me, our boys will have a ready answer if they're ever asked to name their hometown. Stability, lifelong companions, one house, a sense of neighborhood: these we have provided for our offspring. And they resent it all. They are thrill seekers who long for foreign lands and spend their days plotting ways to get the hell outta Dodge. With no irony they criticize me for being provincial, unadventurous, a stick in the mud lacking the gumption or good sense to have raised them in more exotic places. Maybe it's inevitable. The pendulum swings back. Perhaps our boys will raise their families like vagabonds; perhaps our grandchildren will settle down; perhaps that stationary life will incite the next generation of wanderers. We all have a sugar-addicted friend who blames it on her mother's militant refusal to let junk food in the house. She will likely produce a daughter who shops only organic and grows her own sprouts in the kitchen windowsill. The job of parenting is frightening in part because all this back and forth between the generations can feel like a personal slap in the face.

PARENTING CASE STUDY:
The Curse of the Hot Mom

Laura spent childhood embarrassed by her unstylish, overweight mother. Educated, accomplished and devoted to a Girl Power upbringing for her daughters, Mom cultivated an earthy frumpiness that made Laura cringe when they were together in public. In middle school Laura started devising ways to discourage her mother from volunteering at her school or giving rides to her friends. When she became a mother herself—to three beautiful, rambunctious boys—Laura vowed to do the opposite for her brood. She couldn't inform them about makeup and eyebrow tweezing like she might have done with daughters, but she took pride in keeping herself fit and *en vogue*. She remembered envying peers whose parents were at least kind of tuned in to pop culture, so she paid attention to the bands appearing on late night television, thinking she might curb some adolescent resentment with a valiant attempt to stay current. Her sons' friends loved her (naturally) while her kids themselves resented everything about her. Laura did the opposite, all right, but the reaction in her kids was identical. Her appearance made her children cringe when they were together in public.

It's not personal, of course. Why do we strive to provide our children an upbringing different from ours? Because we love them. We want the best for them. We're only trying to protect them from the cruel blows life dealt us and the asinine mistakes we made. The pendulum swings; the earth turns; it's the circle of life. But during the teenage years, parents can try to check our balance by remaining flexible instead of overreacting. Amidst the three-ring circus of raising teenagers, we can seek consistency and some sense of stability by trying to step back from each chaotic situation and ask those three vital questions of ourselves: Do I know what's going on with myself and my family? Must I step in to protect myself or my child from my own emotional reactions? Can I honor my own imperfections and let my children make their own mistakes?

WE'RE STUCK IN THE MIDDLE AGAIN.

As if to rub in the cosmic joke, family dynamics are in perpetual motion. Statistically, parents will experience profound changes to our health and wellbeing while our children are in the throes of adolescence. Menopause and midlife angst are almost guaranteed; other surprises like cancer and diabetes are also likely to rear their ugly heads during these chaotic years. We can, moreover, expect our parents—our children's grandparents—to face major life transformations during these years. When Dorothy Miller (1981) called societal attention to the struggles of the "sandwich generation" she hit the nail on the head. Adults sandwiched between the demands of aging parents and adolescent children are burdened by legal, medical and financial issues as well as complicated, shifting roles within the larger family system.

Nearly everyone I know has a story. A parent dies suddenly and leaves behind a complicated estate and grief-stricken adult children who are smack in the middle of raising teenagers. A grandparent gets sick and requires years of assistance. Elder care is expensive and emotional;

grandparents lash out like angry adolescents when it comes time to relinquish their independence. When Grandma gets sick and lands in ICU, her dutiful daughter drops everything to be at her side. Roles reverse without warning: the daughter suddenly finds herself advocating fulltime for her mom, fighting for care, tapping unknown reserves of strength and gumption. When Mom regains consciousness, her first words are not gratitude or humility, but the usual criticism of her daughter's haircut. These predictable, human patterns—expected during these middle years of our existence—feel so painful and personal, every time!

Grandpa's rapid memory loss causes him to rage about issues long past. His son has a visceral reaction. He is reminded of how much he has disappointed his father over the years and he is frightened by how much his own son might disappoint him. His son's daily and age-appropriate rejection feels like an echo of his father's anger. Once again, parents of teenagers find ourselves stuck between Scylla and Charybdis, raising our families with the devil on one side and the deep blue sea on the other. The aging of America means more resources than ever for those of us sandwiched between the generations and I recommend taking full advantage. If we know what's going on we can seek the advice of those who have moved their parents to assisted living, suffered through the long goodbye of Alzheimer's Disease or shipped their kids off to college and survived. As my parents age and our roles shift, I need to talk honestly about transitions and geriatric care with people who know more than I do. I rely on the camaraderie of my own siblings and the wisdom of specialists, friends, family and bloggers devoted to this straightforward conversation. Even when we know and admit the reality of our situation, however, we are often sandwiched between the tantrums of teenagers and the and vitriol of the elderly. Who can blame Mama Bear for hibernating? On more days than we care to admit—when we are immersed in the painful turbulence of our mutating families—staying in bed seems like the best option. But we know better.

193

WATCH FOR BLIND SPOTS.

Not only do our kids hurt our feelings, they also scare the hell out of us. We fear for their actual lives when they take risks and develop attitudes of apathy or anarchy. But they frighten us most of all when they remind us of ourselves—or not. Whether they're just like us or different in every way, their identity formation stirs the sleeping dragon of our own adolescent angst. If they have interests or talents similar to ours, it's tempting to conflate our experience with theirs. Their teen years may open old wounds or chambers of melancholy in our hearts. We may want to protect them from our mistakes or the side effects of our worst habits; we worry they'll turn into adults as incompetent as we feel. These fears lead us to overreact when the kids are younger and to act pretty kooky when they are adolescents. A mom who was once teased or awkward might defend her beloved child too aggressively on the playground. A dad whose super discipline earned his younger self a starting spot on the team may be too zealous about his athletic child's training regime.

On the other hand, when they are not like us it can be just as confounding. If their passions and choices seem foreign, we fear the chasm between us. The bullied parent may have a terrible time with a child who is aggressive and bossy. The popular jock may be stymied while raising an awkward math geek; the poet-pacifist parents are wounded to the core when their kid joins the Marines. When they remind us of ourselves, it's painful; when they are unlike us they provoke a different (but no less excruciating) set of anxieties. Either way, living with teenagers disturbs the dust on some of the baggage we've kept stored away for many years.

We cannot hope to transform our own struggles unless we seek to recognize them. Parents, as much as we need to know what's really going on with our teenagers, we need to know ourselves. Raising our children can trigger some pretty unpleasant stuff but it can also be an amazing opportunity for us to make peace with ourselves and our pasts. Let us watch for our own blind spots. Let us try to know when our child's journey reminds us of something about ours.

. . . .

PARENTING CASE STUDIES:
The Stage Door and the Driving Range

1. Here's one from my own personal files. I wouldn't wish an actor's life on my worst enemy. I loved my years in theatre school and living like a pauper in Manhattan but it's a difficult profession. Like the cliché I am, I left it all behind (all that glamorous auditioning and waitressing and starving) to start a family. It was with mixed feelings, then, that I agreed to sign my son up for the Saturday acting class he wanted to take. I was reluctant to agree when the class led very quickly to a series of professional acting jobs for him. Before we knew it, my husband and I stepped into the role of manager-driver for a boy with a career I had only dreamed about for myself. Often the irony hit me when I dropped him off at the stage door or graded student essays outside a rehearsal hall. Here I was reporting to the theatre every night for half-hour call, just as I had once imagined I'd do. Here I was supporting (in my way) the development of new works on the American stage, as I had intended. Every opening night I was there: in the audience. I was walking the steps of my former journey, but it had nothing whatever to do with me and I knew it. It was easy to be proud of my boy; it was difficult not be envious of his success. A few years later the satire of my life came full-circle on a girls' trip back to my old stomping grounds in New York City. My bestie and I ducked into a live-music venue to see friends perform (friends we knew because they had shared various stages with my son). The show was starting

195

as we made our way to the bar, feeling *tres* bohemian and fancy-free. I waved a greeting and was warmly welcomed from the stage: "All right, everybody! Augie's mom, in the house!" Not Lisa, not any of the cool nicknames I earned in my twenties, not actor, performer, writer or even woman-about-town . . . Augie's Mom. There. In the City. Where I had once been legendary in my own mind. Way to rub it in, Universe. Way to confirm those late night fears about my very Self, consumed or snuffed out by the endless demands of my offspring.

2. Our friend Scott's grand passion is golf, but he has rarely played a round in his life without hearing his father's voice in his head. He is haunted by impressions of golf as self-indulgent, a lazy man's game, just this side of wickedness. Every pleasant afternoon on the links is tainted by a nagging sense he should be working, doing something productive, making something of himself. At the same time, he mourns the player he might have been with any measure of support behind him. One gift Scott has worked hard to give his children is frequent and guilt-free access to the sport he loves. He can't provide exotic trips to destination courses, but he has found affordable ways for them to take lessons and play. The kids have been mostly willing but they get frustrated by the concentration and civility required of the game. As his 10-year-old once explained, "You know us, Dad; we like to jump around." Of course, Scott trusts his investment of time, money and range tokens will pay off eventually, but he dies a little every time his teenagers turn down a chance to play. He is conscious not to force his passion down their throats, but when his offspring show signs of raw talent, it is crazy hard not to push just a little. When they choose pool parties with

their friends over tournaments, Scott is a little crushed. Each time they shrug off an invitation to join him on the practice green, he tries not to concentrate on the wasted opportunity. He tries to trust the process—golf is a lifelong pastime, after all—and keep his feelings of resentment at bay. He tries not to say things like, "If my dad had ever asked me . . ." and, "If I had been given this chance when I was your age . . . ." He tries not to use words such as "ungrateful" or "spoiled." He tries. But it is really, really hard.

· ·

If we stay aware of these crazy (but predictable) patterns of family life, we may more eagerly know when teenage troubles hit our particularly sensitive nerves. If we make regular, concerted attempts to admit our own vulnerabilities, we can work on disentangling ourselves from our children and their unique process of growing up. Best of all, if we stay detached and work on transforming our own pain, we can set a good example for our kids. I've seen it happen in families and I have marveled at the positive results. A parent who lights a candle instead of cursing the darkness, who tells the truth, who takes a stand or forgives an enemy, can lead the way to generations of transformation. I know you'll want to punch me as I remind you again of the fine line (but I must). Letting our teenagers into too much of our struggle can be as dangerous as denying it. We seek a balance, as always: between being honest and burdening them with our truth, between setting an example and setting unreasonable expectations. Parenting, of course, is complicated and it's hard to fully practice detachment or let the teenage years roll off us like water from a duck's back. But we can try. And in trying, we make a difference. As we seek to know our teenagers and ourselves, we can check for the blind spots that awaken our own demons and prevent us from being the best parents we can be.

197

STEP INTO THE FEAR.

I have learned from my own parenting and from my research that when something about our kid scares us, that thing needs attention. Sometimes it's a conversation we think we need to have with our kid that scares us (because we have discovered paraphernalia or condoms or violent poetry). We may dance around the topic, employ euphemisms or make jokes, but we avoid a forthright *tête-à-tête*. Often we practice the fine art of denial and tell our gut to hush; everything's just fine. Usually, we are afraid: of the truth, the consequences, the scene that will follow, our child's anger, our own failure. Listen up, Folks, because this is 100%: the exact thing that frightens you—the conversation or confrontation or whatever it is—is exactly the thing that needs to happen. Fear is like a gift from Mother Nature if we accept it: a kick in the gut, an alarm, a warning bell. When we know the blind spots threatening our parenting efforts, we can face them, transform them and find our balance on the high wire. It ain't easy, but your kids are worth it and so are you. If it scares you, it's important. Step into that fear.

Chapter Twenty-One

(Protect Yourself)
Oxygen Masks, Tightropes and
the Wisdom of Your Tribe

IT IS NOT uncommon to hear developmental experts turn to aviation for inspiration, describing how parents navigate the "flight plan" of family life. Some of the worst, most debilitating turbulence hits during the adolescent years. To extend the metaphor, think of a flight attendant's safety speech: "If you are traveling with a child or someone who requires assistance," we are reminded, "secure your oxygen mask first, before you assist the other person." During our children's adolescence, parents need to do the same. We need to find a way to stay healthy and keep ourselves sane in order to care for our still-growing, exhausting, mercurial kids. If we think back to our tightrope walker, we recall a similar lesson.

Imagine you're walking an actual tightrope. You have your own arms to stretch out and help you balance. You rely on core strength. If you tighten those abs, concentrate and place your feet carefully, you stay upright! Thanks to great focus and internal strength, you even learn to juggle up there. You're asked to move into the center ring and do the death-defying stunt of tightrope walking with another acrobat riding on your shoulders. You and your new partner will have to practice this maneuver. You'll do so for hours on a tumbling mat, wearing pads and head protection. There will be a lot of give and take between you as you rehearse the weight exchange and learn how your bodies move best together. Eventually you'll develop a wordless rapport and work together in harmony, in tandem, on your show-stopping act.

When you're the parent of a teenager, your performing partner is distinctly less willing. The human being selected to perch artfully on your shoulders does not play by the basic rules of tumbling or circus arts. An adolescent person may instead body slam himself into you. She may grab onto your ankles while you are trying to walk. Perhaps you've got a half-willing partner who will climb onto your shoulders, but while sitting there, he'll also cover your eyes and wiggle and squirm and shoot hoops into an imaginary net. On the metaphor of the tightrope and in real life, it feels like teenagers are trying to destroy us.

We have to take care of ourselves. We have to put the oxygen mask on ourselves first before we can help our kids or our families. We know this. It's a cultural phenomenon. We make furtive attempts and lots of New Years' resolutions to be less stressed and healthier. I hope the oxygen mask and tightrope walker will remind you why it's not selfish to take care of yourself. By now, you know my stance on staying vigilant while raising teenagers (I'm all for it). Self-care does not mean abandoning our kids or checking out during these vulnerable decades. I've given you some new role models who practice healthy, daily habits and make the best of living with adolescent people. As tempted as we are to medicate the chaos of our lives with unhealthy choices, few of us can deny the benefits of exercise, communication and eating well. We should give ourselves a break and a good, stiff drink now and then, but to meet the challenges of Teenage Wasteland we need to stay frosty, be in good shape and have our wits about us. Whatever it means to you—a meditation room or a long weekly bath with a good novel or getting medical attention or eating fewer donuts because they make you feel sick—I hope you'll try to protect yourself and stay as healthy as you can.

SEEK THE COUNSEL OF ELDERS.

As you are also aware by now, I believe it's important to seek the counsel and comfort of those who have walked the path ahead of us. Once again, I remind you to find strength in your community, in other people, in parents whose kids took them through hell but who came out okay. Talk to them. First of all (as I have pointed out a time or two), their sense of humor will comfort you. When you're in knots over your 16-year-old's choice of a romantic companion, your friends whose kids are now 30 will say simple things like, "Oh, that won't last." Problem solved. Secondly, older parents can help by telling you how they got through it all. They'll tell you things they did and things they wish they had done. It's nice getting advice from fellow travelers on this brutal road who can help us gain a new vantage point, a new perspective. How we see can set us free! [2]

Chapter Twenty-Two

(Honor Yourself)
Gut Checks, Parenting Peer Pressure and Staying on Course

THERE IS NOT one job description for the vocation of raising a family; there are too many. I recall being shocked at how many books it took to birth a baby. Shortly after that joyful pee-on-a-stick moment, my husband I rushed dutifully to our local bookstore and stood overwhelmed in the Pregnancy and Birth section. I recall feeling dizzy as my eyes went up, then to the left and the right: as far as I could see, tomes on healthy eating habits, prenatal exercise and the perils of crib bumpers. Should we ever doubt the cultural importance middle America puts on parenting, let us spend an hour amongst these endless shelves filled with "expert" advice on the subject (this very book included, of course).

The proliferation of parenting counsel in all forms (blogs and websites, television programming, workshops, support groups) underscores another important cultural conviction: we may feel ill-equipped and we may not know our job description, but we think parenting *matters*. Parents believe we can make a difference in the development of our offspring. And we are not wrong. Everything we do, say and think has a profound and lasting effect on our children. Societies across the world agree on the basic value of protecting, nurturing and speaking to babies and little kids. Adults tend to believe—with variances informed by culture, resources or personality—in the importance of preparing children for a growing series of responsibilities and commitments. By and large, we understand the family as part economic unit and part support system. In every case I have ever experienced, parents want the very best for their children. But the differences in how we interpret our roles is a complicated amalgam of our family backgrounds and our own identity formation. It takes a village to raise a child, but the villagers don't agree on much of anything, including what the heck they're doing.

Parents of teenagers need to stay flexible and ready to pivot. It's tempting to lean into societal pressures and into our kids: their lives, dramas, struggles, passions and fears. If we lean too far, they will pull us right off the tightrope. In this incredible balancing act, it is best—like the tightrope walker—to focus on our own bodies and stay upright. Which means before we let our kids throw us off balance with the details of their lives, we take care of our own. When teenagers or other parents talk nonsense, we remember our role models who teach detachment and patience. We take the higher road because we are the grown ups. And certainly we resist peer pressure. I mean, we're not the teenagers . . . right?

. . . .

PARENTING CASE STUDY:
The Tale of Two Water Bottles

I remember feeling like a terrible parent one summer afternoon at a soccer field. After running around like maniacs for half an hour, our tiny athletes came panting to the sidelines for a break. I handed my boys a baggie of cashews, a couple of grapes and the water bottles I'd filled that morning, now lukewarm. Suddenly, we were surrounded by teammates sipping from similar bottles, but their water was miraculously ice cold. Thus I discovered the invention of a new and exciting product: ice trays designed specifically for sport bottles. Available at fine stores everywhere, this fabulous innovation produced thin cylinders of ice which slid easily into narrow necks of water bottles.

I knew in an instant I would never be the kind of mother who made such a purchase. I knew I would never remember to fill the special trays, nor take the time to deposit the clever tubes of ice into bottles before leaving the house. (I won't even go into how my snacks compared to the adorable, organic *bento* boxes produced by the other mothers. I can only handle one parenting deficit at a time.) On a certain level, I realized my priorities—and my tolerance of tepid beverages—were different than many of my peers. I trusted my love, value and support of my children, but on another level I felt guilty and lazy for not ensuring a 24-hour optimal temperature for their drinking water. It sounds silly now, but honest to God, those new-fangled ice cube trays made me feel like everyone was doing it better than I was.

A few summers later, I threw all our water bottles into the trash. Hysteria about the potential effects of BPAs in hard plastics was at a fever pitch in our circle of parents and friends. More than I worried about adverse effects on my children's health, I feared the judgmental stares of other mothers. By this time, I understood the spectrum of parenting agendas. I knew some of my family's choices—the music to which we exposed our kids, our fluid concept of bedtime, my indulgence of noise and mess—stood in opposition to many of our friends. I felt mostly okay with the quality of our family's life and the health of our children and I confess I didn't really care much about the dangers of BPAs. It just seemed important to play by *some* of the rules, so as not to call attention to the depth of my parenting insufficiencies. It was hard not to worry my children would be socially shunned because their neglectful mother let them drink out of poison bottles.

. . . .

I know. This is nuts. And it's only the tip of the iceberg. We all know parenting isn't a competitive sport. We nod our heads when priests, prophets and best friends prompt us to let go of our need for perfection. Raising a family is a messy process. We know this. We should forgive ourselves and do our best, we repeat. Enjoy the moment; choose joy; be grateful for all we have. Yet despite our attempts at freeing ourselves from expectations, one Pinterest image of an organized closet, smiling family vacation or "professionally styled" birthday party can knock us right off our game. I am down on my knees begging you once again to forgive yourself for being a less than perfect parent. Please consult our new role models who help us take a new look at the tough job of being gentle to ourselves and our offspring. Try to remember most other parents feel as overwhelmed and incompetent as we do. No matter how it looks, the reality is this: most of us are too busy second-guessing ourselves and feeling ragged from family chaos to pay much attention to anyone else's water bottles.

Society has come to only a vague consensus on the goals of parenting. We seek to equip the next generation with tools for the physical, economic and psychosocial demands of the adult world but few of us share identical visions of the toolbox. Even happily married spouses have different assumptions about parenting; the water is further muddied by the expectations of neighbors, friends, teachers, experts and mommy bloggers. Don't get me wrong: I am a huge fan of open family systems and community parenting. I would be lost without the opinions, help and belief systems of those who comprise my village. But it's confusing from the start, all the passionate and wildly divergent opinions on pacifiers, transitional objects, screen time and sleep patterns. Meanwhile, we are unfortunately prone to questioning our own parenting and feeling inadequate. It's important, especially during the teenage years, to trust your gut. To resist peer pressure. To stay centered so you and your family can honor your unique journey and do what's best for all of you.

PARENTING CASE STUDY:
Insult to Injury

Jane stretched on the living room floor and congratulated herself. Dinner was in the crock pot; Daddy was driving carpool; she had squeezed in a nice run after work. Jane inhaled deeply, felt her spine sink into the floor, relished the moment of peace. As she lifted her hips into the bridge position, her calm was disrupted by the sudden appearance of her 12-year-old son. He screamed in horror: "Oh my God, Mom! What are you *doing*?" He wheeled around, ran into the bathroom and slammed the door, leaving Jane bewildered on the carpet. I know for a fact when this kid was little he viewed his mother with unconditional love and compassion. Like most of us, Jane relished a few blissful years of seeing herself through her child's eyes—imperfections and scars and everything—and knowing she was whole and perfect and worthy. Now, the look of disgust on his prepubescent face reactivated every single body-image insecurity she developed during her own adolescence.

Here is just one more example of how difficult our job is. As we endeavor to stay neutral and mentally healthy, teenagers will bitch-slap us right out of any sense of enlightenment we might have enjoyed, ever. In a thousand ways, our teenagers make the job of parenting impossible. We might start believing them as they work to convince us they don't need us anymore. Out of exhaustion or wounded pride, we check out. We give up on them. We get embroiled in their adolescent drama or stung by their rebellious words. We are exhausted from all this parenting and it is much, much easier to take a nap in a dark room than it is to sleep with one eye open for the next several years. But if we remain vigilant and dedicated to loving them just as we did when they were toddlers, we help them negotiate their final steps toward growing up.

Poor Jane on the living room floor! Part of the reason her son freaked out, of course, was his sudden, nascent awareness of his mother's sexuality. *Gross*, right? To the son it feels like she has changed and he hates her for it and the whole thing straight-up wigs him out. Change on the home front makes adolescents feel untethered. Middle school kids might despise us when we redecorate the living room; no matter how fantastic the improvements, they are unnerved by the change. They likewise resent it if we shave our beards, wear a new cut of jeans or take up a new hobby. Teenagers count on us for consistency.

Wait. Don't they condemn and reject that very consistency and any form of rules or boundaries? Yes. Yes, they do. And therein lies just one cruel joke in the epic comedy of raising teenagers. They crave and reject boundaries equally. It is also interesting to note how much our vulnerability bums out our kids. For some, it begins when they are actual toddlers. Sometimes when we are weak, sad or injured, exhausted or sick, our children act less sympathetic than angry. A three-year-old might throw a tantrum because Mommy's walking pneumonia makes her voice sounds like a dinosaur. Once my own child punched me in the stomach because I was crying after a mild argument with his father. The same child regularly brought me breakfast in bed and kissed my boo-boos. He was not void of compassion and he was often sweet. But my genuine display of vulnerability left him more vulnerable than he could stand. He lashed out in anger and because he was five it was kind of funny. When a teenager does the same or the equivalent, it's scary and dangerous. The worst part, obviously, is that often we are vulnerable in direct relationship to them. At least 70 percent of my bad days are caused by my offspring, who are in turn annoyed and frightened by the fact that I have bad days. They say awful things when we are at our worst; they push us away when we could really use a hug. As we know, one great way to survive the storms of adolescence is to remain neutral and detached. Their outbursts have relatively little to do with us. Their rage is not our rage; our ideas are not theirs; they want different things than we do because we are different people. It's best to try not to let teenagers rock your boat, no matter how much they've caused the storm. It's hard to do. It's exhausting and inconvenient. But remaining calm and forgiving ourselves is a good vantage from which to raise adolescents.

My Friends, you've got this. I'm asking you to do difficult things, staying vigilant and taking care of your teenagers and yourselves, but you've got everything it takes. This process—this three-ring circus of family disruption—is natural, normal and necessary. It's painful and it feels personal but it's not permanent. I hope these stories and these tools for parenting will help you feel less alone and more apt to share your struggles with your tribe. I hope you will take parenting time outs and ask the three most important questions of raising teenagers. I hope you will find some balance and remember to laugh at yourself. No matter how chaotic and crazy things get, you are exactly the parent your children need. They're lucky to have you. And someday—*inshallah*—their brains will fully develop and you'll recognize them again and they might even thank you for being there for them during the storms of adolescence. We live in hope. We all shine on!

> Why in the world are we here?
> Surely not to live in pain and fear . . .
> Well, we all shine on
> Like the moon and the stars and the sun
> Yeah, we all shine on . . .
>
> ~John Lennon

Endnotes

1 (Page 29) I hope the idea of a perfect parent makes you laugh out loud. Accepting imperfection in our teenagers and ourselves is vital to surviving the three-ring circus of parenting. I don't even like to use labels such as "good" or "bad" in regard to parents. Surely we can give ourselves (and each other) a break, trust that we all have pure intentions and we're all honestly doing the best we can. Some parents, though—the ones I admire and try to emulate—maintain that elusive balance on the high wire and seem to survive a little more intact than the rest of us.

Psychologists who study parenting styles—led by the work of Diana Baumrind (1991) give us the authoritative parent as an ideal model. Authoritative parents are strict, consistent and loving. Rather than focusing on an idealized version of their children or external, absolute standards, authoritative parents adjust their expectations to the needs of the person. They model rational decision making and listen to their children's arguments, but reserve the right to make final decisions. They communicate, explain, and administer consistent, logical consequences. Authoritative parents believe in the rights of children to be respected and have their own needs met. During adolescence, these parents teach and guide their children. Most importantly, they try to help growing children learn to balance their responsibility to society with their individual needs and desires. Authoritative parents tend to produce adults with better self-esteem and sense of purpose. They strike a balance in parenting that allows teenagers to express—and become—their own unique people with an interior sense of right, wrong, dignity and identity.

2 (Page 68 & 201): How You See Can Set You Free! I believe in this concept so much I wrote a book about it. Envisioned by my dear friend Rita Mailander, *Bella Bug Says, "Let Me See!"* is a vividly illustrated lesson for children (and all of us) on how to maintain a positive world view. When Bella Bug gets stuck in a rut, a crew of friends helps her remember to see things differently. Available on amazon.com and iBooks.

3 (Page 154): I lately heard a brand-new Mama complain about her mother's and grandmother's friends and their eager requests to see the little one. "I don't want a bunch of old ladies passing my baby around like a football," she said. I withered inside. I didn't say anything to her because every new family has a right to their own morays. But I thought to myself, "What a silly, shortsighted thing to say. Do you know what those old ladies are doing? They're welcoming your child to Life! You lucky thing! They're communicating love and safety and a sense of belonging. They also know more than you do and they're coming to help you. They're promising to be there for you and your family! Girl, you can't do this *without* a bunch of old ladies who pass your baby around like a football!" I didn't say it, but I believe it's true. What's more, the older parents who want to hold the infant (and play with the toddler) quite likely need a dose of innocence. Whether they have adolescents or grown children, their kids don't smell fresh and adorable anymore. I beg new Mamas to share children with the community because it's good for parents, kids and the elders who need a baby hug every now and again. Same goes for parents of older kids. We need the tribe!

4 (Page 171): Karen Dawson Haag is an educator and champion of literacy, which might explain her particular brand of brilliance. Please check out, learn from and use her websites, www.liketowrite.com (a free resource for passionate people about helping students write well) and www.liketoread.com (a free resource for passionate people about helping children enjoy reading).

Sources Cited

Baumrind, D. (1991). *Effective parenting during the early adolescent transition*. Family Transitions. Cowan, P.A. and Hetherington, M., ed. Laurence Erlbaum Associates, Hillsdale, NJ.

Goldstein, J. (2011). *A secular trend toward earlier male sexual maturity: Evidence from shifting ages of male young adult mortality*. PLOSOne. Accessed July 6, 2015: http://journals.plos.org/plosone/article?id=10.1371/journal.pone.0014826

Miller, D.A. (1981). *The 'sandwich' generation: adult children of the aging*. Social Work; 26 (5): 419-423. doi: 10.1093/sw/26.5.419

Miller, L., & Spiegel, A. (Hosts). (2015, January 23). *How to become batman*. Invisiblia [Audio Podcast]. Retrieved from http://www.npr.org/programs/invisibilia/378577902/how-to-become-batman.

Rousseau, J. (1762). *Emile, or education*. Trans. B. Foxley. (1921) E.P. Dutton, New York, NY.

Steinberg, L. D. (2014). *Age of opportunity: Lessons from the new science of adolescence*. Houghton Mifflin Harcourt, New York, NY.

Wiggins, G. P., McTighe, J., Kiernan, L. J., Frost, F., & Association for Supervision and Curriculum Development. (1998). *Understanding by design*. Association for Supervision and Curriculum Development, Alexandria, VA.

About the Author

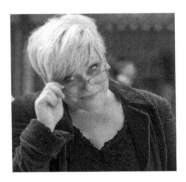

LISA LANE FILHOLM earned her B.A. (English Literature) from Colorado College, her M.Ed. (Curriculum and Instruction) from the University of Colorado-Denver, and her professional actor training credentials at Trinity Rep Conservatory in Providence, RI. She has published two children's books and has written, edited and served as spokesperson for a variety of freelance and contract clients.

Made in the USA
San Bernardino, CA
17 August 2017